Praise for *Bonjour, Bonjour, Breast Cancer—I'm Still Smiling!*

Witty and serious, fun and rigorous, this book is exactly what the doctor (and psychologist) would prescribe! *Bonjour, Breast Cancer—I'm Still Smiling!* can be a life changing and life affirming gift to any cancer patient and to anyone else afflicted by physical or psychological illness.

— Tal Ben-Shahar, best-selling author of
Happier and *Choose the Life You Want*

The beauty of this book is that a person doesn't need to have breast cancer to learn and incorporate the wisdom that Princess Diane imparts. It is truly a guidebook for survival. A person facing a diagnosis of any disease or condition that has turned that person's world upside down can take her words to heart, act on them, and come out seeing with new eyes and smiling with refreshed optimism. I am a primary care physician and will be recommending this book to many as they try to find ways to manage their conditions and emotions to a better sense of wellbeing.

— Teresa M Schaer, MD, Internist and Geriatrician,
Signature Health Solutions

I'll be honest: I don't like cancer. More honesty: I really do like breasts. All the honesty: The only way I can even think about breast cancer is through the genuine, inspirational, positive, and above all, funny words of Princess Diane von Brainisfried. Whether you think you need this book or not, you do. It's a comforting guide on the road trip to the rest of your life. Read it!

—Jeff Kreisler, comedian, speaker, and bestselling author
of *Dollars and Sense* and *Get Rich Cheating*

Diane strikes the perfect notes! She is a comfort and inspiration to anyone diagnosed with breast cancer and anyone who is helping someone through it. She packs the humor of our humanity with practical information to navigate this all-too-common disease. In truth, there is inspiration for everyone. By sharing her journey, Diane taps into her power and can help any of us tap into ours. When we do that, we are in alignment and make smart choices that bring personal happiness. This is a book you will want to own.

—Ellen Berenholz, Founder, Executive Director Pagus: Africa

The Princess's book is an emotional roller-coaster journey and romp of a breast cancer survivor, written as if personally talking to you— which is an art form. It is a romp partly because of its positivity, soul, humor, fear, spirituality, synchronicity in the universe, family, friends, sleepovers, optimism, the gift of now and being "hoit" and bald. All delicately, embracingly discussed. This book is for navigating life's difficulties and triumphs of the spirit with awareness, and it should be shared with those close and far.

—Calvin Schwartz, Senior Writer, Producer, co-host, NJ Discover.com

I have always labeled myself as "Pollyanna." When our house burned, I saw it as a decorating opportunity. When my father was dying, it brought me and my siblings together. But when I had my breast cancer scare (and I was fortunate—it was only a scare), I felt my world spinning out of control. My wonderful husband offered to leave work, but I said no. If he came, it would have made the in-office biopsy too real. So I sat stoically alone while they prepared me for the procedure. As I left the doctor's office, an older gentleman was walking up the stairs. He must have seen the barely concealed panic on my face and asked if I was okay. I looked at him and asked the perfect stranger for a hug. I will never forget that hug or the kindness this stranger shared with me. *Bonjour, Breast Cancer—I'm Still Smiling!* is a wonderful hug. I smiled, laughed, cried, and cheered. We are indeed in the presence of a gracious, kind princess.

—Michelle Schaap, Esq., CIPP/US, Member,
Chiesa Shahinian & Giantomasi PC

This book is brilliant, witty, poignant, profound, funny, inspiring, and so well written. I absolutely love how Princess Diane weaves psychological theory and research with personal stories and meaningful quotes and allegories. She made me laugh out loud, cry, and think. She's a warrior, and this book is powerfully optimistic!

—Hannah Bubis, President, Cre8MediaHub

In her book *Bonjour, Breast Cancer—I'm Still Smiling!*, the message and meaning received from Diane's wit, courage, humor, and honesty provide a fresh guts-and-grace look into what it means to be touched by unexpected breast cancer. The down and up are all part of the process. Having a guide to help you ride the waves, honestly think, imagine and see things differently, feel your truth, and smell and taste the edges of the terrifying moments of choice when there is no clear path is something anyone dealing with breast cancer will benefit from. Diane shows us a new way to show up for life, no matter what shows up!

—Debbie Rosas, Founder of Nia Technique Movement Art

Bonjour, Breast Cancer– I'm Still Smiling!

Bonjour, Breast Cancer– I'm Still Smiling!

Wit, Wisdom, and Optimism for Beating the Breast Cancer Blues

Princess Diane von Brainisfried

Bonjour, Breast Cancer—I'm Still Smiling!
Wit, Wisdom, and Optimism for Beating the Breast Cancer Blues
by Princess Diane von Brainisfried

This book is part memoir, and I have tried to recreate events, locales and conversations from my memories of them. In order to protect their privacy, in some instances I have changed the names and characteristics of individuals and places, and I may have changed some details.

ISBN: 978-1-7326586-0-8 (Print)
ISBN: 978-1-7326586-1-5 (eBook)
LCCN: 2019906275

HarMaxi Productions, LLC
1560 Van Buren Drive
North Brunswick, New Jersey 08902

Editing by Melanie Mulhall, Dragonheart, DragonheartWritingandEditing.com
Book Design by Nick Zelinger, NZ Graphics, NZGraphics.com

First Edition
Printed in the United States of America

With profound gratitude, I dedicate this book, and my happy heart, to my mother, Geraldine Prose Young, MD, and father (now in heaven), Irving Young, MD, for their unconditional love, endless encouragement, and invaluable guidance. They never—and I mean never—rained on my parade.

Contents

INTRODUCTION

If you want to be happy, don't focus on what's crappy.
–Princess Diane von Brainisfried

*B*onjour, my royal friends. Welcome to my kingdom! I'm Princess Diane von Brainisfried, and I'm absolutely thrilled to meet you. If you're reading this and you've been diagnosed with breast cancer, I take my tiara off to you. Not everyone has the courage to follow where the smiles live during challenging times. But you do, and the proof is in the *crème brûlée*—because you're here.

This whole breast cancer thing can deflate a person's mental state faster than a balloon in a Cutco knife factory. It's one big, sloppy fear sandwich with a side order of cries. I should know. I'm a breast cancer survivor, or as I like to say, breast cancer *aliver*. But help is here.

I'm going to share some things that I hope will help you handle the breast cancer journey with positivity, optimism, soulfulness, and humor to help you become a Bonjour-Breast-Cancer-I'm-Still-Smiling princess too. You will discover strategies I used to self-help myself back to seeing my goblet half full and put the ha-has and hallelujahs back into my life.

I'll let you in on a little secret. I've been told by many people that I laugh too much. That's like saying my wallet is too fat, my palace has too many loos, my puns are too groan-worthy, my teeth are too white, my dog is too well-behaved, or I've won too many screenplay and musical awards. That's why I don't give a rat's ring finger what anyone thinks about my laughter habits. Studies have shown that laughter fosters health and healing. Who's laughing now?

I don't have a pie-in-the-sky treatise, although who doesn't like a slice of pie now and then? I realized pretty quickly that I had no frame of reference for handling a diagnosis of breast cancer. Nothing prepares you for this stuff. *Where the heck do I put my mind? How do I keep my happiness equilibrium? How do I not sink into despair? How do I not get swallowed up in fear?* These were the thoughts that came to me in the first few minutes after diagnosis. Never mind the deluge that came in the following hours and days.

Fortunately, I'm a Certified Positive Psychology Life Coach. What's cool about the field of positive psychology is that it's more about identifying and building on what is working in your life rather than what isn't working so well. The field of positive psychology also includes the study of optimism and how to learn and adopt traits common among optimists.

Why is cultivating an optimistic attitude important? For one thing, optimists tend to be more resilient, a critical asset for weathering life's "slings and arrows of outrageous fortune," as some bard with a shaky spear used to say. And there are a whole lot more perks that optimists tend to enjoy, such as better health, less stress, and greater happiness. Looks like optimism is one hard-working, multi-purpose happiness household spray.

Lest you feel disheartened because you're pretty certain that if you Google the word *pessimist*, you'll find your picture, take heart. Research shows optimism can be learned. And if you feel you don't want to become more optimistic because you think optimists aren't realists, put your worries in the compost heap and put a big yellow sticky on this fact: It's not that optimists are blind to the reality of the tough stuff they're facing, it's just that they find a way to look at difficult events in the best light that they can. As I like to say, name it, reframe it, and *then* claim it, princess.

And you guys out there, listen up. Although what I have to share is geared to my sister princesses, I know that breast cancer is not an exclusively female club. Many guys have ridden in this rodeo. If you are a guy or identify as a guy, the positivity and optimism strategies I'm going to offer will be a big help to you as well. Just skim the parts that don't resonate while sticking your fingers in your ears and chanting "Nanny, nanny, poo, poo."

Handling the panic and fear surrounding my breast cancer diagnosis was one of the biggest challenges of my life. The good news is, I found my way back to a happy heart. Now I wake up every morning and say, "Bonjour, breast cancer—I'm still smiling!" And you can too! I want to help you adopt a positive, optimistic, one-foot-in-front-of-the-other, steady-as-she-goes attitude like I did so the journey doesn't have to be *so* scary.

Finding your way to a happy headspace may not happen overnight. It sure didn't for me. But your *decision* to look for a way to the happy headspace, to lean into that direction, *can* happen in an instant. For me, it took a hefty dose of desire, followed by finding and implementing practical strategies for positivity. I'm happier than a pig in a kosher deli to share these strategies with you.

Before I continue, you might be wondering who this Princess Diane von Brainisfried is and where she came from. I was waiting for you to ask. I was born inside a Tiffany box, bottle-fed on Coco (Chanel), and weaned on karats. I only recently learned of my royal roots when I discovered a coat of arms on my father's side of the closet. But I assure you, I got the legs from my mother's side.

When I'm not smashing champagne bottles over the bows of ships or blogging my brains out at my palace desk, I'm an attorney-turned-motivational speaker and Certified Positive Psychology Life Coach. I've won awards for my screenplays and musicals, I blog, and I'm an opera singer. I'm also a Francophile. Hence the big Eiffel Tower on my cheek. And if you think I might tend to be just a little hoity-toity wife with all that on top of my princess status, the fact that I'm a wife, mother of two large land animals called boys, and *grand-mère* to a small one keeps me appropriately humble—but no less optimistic.

Before my diagnosis of breast cancer, I had already embarked on a mission to help people thrive happily through my "How to Be Royally Happy" workshops, lectures, and posts from my palace desk. I never thought I would write about my breast cancer experience. When I was first diagnosed, my brilliant (as in genius-grade) brother encouraged me to write about it, but I totally nixed the idea. At the time, I could more imagine writing about the highs and lows of hemorrhoids than the trajectory of my breast cancer experience. I just wanted to put my head down, plough through, and put the whole crap sandwich in the compost heap behind me. I couldn't imagine wanting to relive even one second. I didn't want to deal with phantom pain.

But then something interesting happened. As I faced each challenge, I was finding ways to handle it with positivity, optimism, humor, and spirituality. That's the thing about breast cancer—it tends to bring out the best in us. You'll see. We just have to dig deep. We've got to do what the golfer Junnah in *The Legend of Bagger Vance* tells young Hardy. Hardy is a kid of about ten, and he's embarrassed that his daddy is sweeping streets during the Great Depression. He feels it's beneath his father's dignity. Junnah explains to Hardy that his daddy has more dignity than all of the others because instead of declaring bankruptcy like everyone else, he stared down adversity and did battle with it.

It took some time, but after the initial shock wore off, the real me kicked back in. The me who loves life. The me who is silly and loves to have fun. The me with the overactive imagination who sees magic in upside-down rainbows and makes wishes on dandelions. The me who laughs so much she's sometimes mistaken for a hyena—except when sporting a tiara. Seriously, who ever saw a hyena sporting a tiara?

I knew I would forget what I was learning if I didn't write it down. And for my own sake, I didn't want to lose what I was learning. But after a while, I realized that the wisdom I was gaining was a precious gift I could share with others for finding happiness in adversity and for experiencing accelerated personal growth. I started feeling compelled—actually called—to a higher duty to share what I learned with you. Thus, I sat down at my palace desk and started jotting down all the discoveries that helped make my daily ups and downs more up than down.

Look, it's not easy to be Ms. Jolly Holly Hoot'n Holler when it feels like you've got a bull's-eye target on your head. But despite the many aspects of breast cancer that can cause dismay, there's so much *good* you can find on this journey, so much soulful discovery, so much room for positive transformation, so much learning to wake up and smell the roses, so much possibility to help others through what you learn that you may create greater meaning in your life and end up seeing this breast cancer "gig" as a gift! That's what happened to me. Princess's honor.

One of my goals is to empower you to move beyond feeling like a victim of breast cancer to feeling like you've stepped into your own power more completely than ever before. I found strategies for happiness and optimism that helped me not only cope but thrive—strategies that helped me regain and maintain my happiness equilibrium. I'm going to arm *you* with the same tools that I used to grab life by the "Balzac" and live the royally happy life that we all deserve, in spite of the darn diagnosis. I can't make your cancer diagnosis and all that it entails go away, but I can help you find ways to make the experience all a whole lot better. And maybe even better than ever. That's how it was for me.

If you or someone you know has been diagnosed with breast cancer and could use some powerful and practical advice for facing the challenges ahead, including how to find your happiness mojo and remain—or become—optimistic about life, you're in the right palace . . . I mean place. I'm going to scoop you up into my heart and hold your hand while I walk you step-by-step through my experiences. I'll show you tons of different strategies that worked for me to help me restore my equilibrium and stoke my joy of life, and I hope you don't mind that I serve it up with a little silliness while we're at it. Bye-bye, palace pop-up pity party! *Welcome to your best new life!*

Optimism is one hard-working
multipurpose happiness household spray.

1

The Magic of Seeing
with New Eyes

If I let cancer steal my joy, then I will have died while I'm still alive.
–Princess Diane von Brainisfried

I've always considered myself to be a happy, upbeat, optimistic person. I've been told I have a sunny disposition. Rather recently, a distant, elderly relative met me for the second time in his life and said, "I know *you*, you're giggle girl!"

Of course, even though I'm a princess, I'm still human. I can sink into a murky-watered, alligator-infested moat like the best of 'em. But the key is, I opt not to stay there, and I use my positivity strategies as a lifeline to pull myself out.

After breast cancer banged on my palace front door knocker, I worried that this was going to be a game changer. I initially wondered how a princess could be happy and optimistic in the face of such a shocking trauma and the fear and uncertainty that flowed from it. I wondered if I was going to have to turn in my positive psychology life coach badge.

It took a little time, but I finally shook off those thoughts like a wet dog in front of a warm hearth. I took a mental deep dive to figure out how to handle being sucker punched by breast cancer. I had to find the solution to my cancer conundrum so my life wouldn't be robbed of joy in whatever time I had left. Breast cancer, bite me! The writer Marcel Proust famously stated, "The voyage of discovery is not in seeking new landscapes, but in having new eyes." I had to find a way to see things with new eyes.

I did. I even wrote a poem about it—well, and about butterflies and cow pies.

Butterflies and Cow Pies and Seeing with New Eyes

The butterfly unfolds
At caterpillar's end,
Breathtaking to behold
Rebirth, and beauty's friend.

As cows unfurl their poop
In mounds bedecked by flies,
When dashed beneath some boot
The dung becomes cow pies.

Likewise, we'll rise to meet
Our challenges, and thrive,
Turn sour into sweet
By seeing with new eyes.

I once had a yoga teacher who told us, "It's not what is happening to you that's important, it's what you tell yourself is happening to you that's important." I thought she was beyond cool. She was a breast cancer survivor who had kept one breast and had the other removed. She didn't have any reconstruction, so when she wore a tank top, the absence of one breast was obvious. She exuded the essence of take-me-as-I-am self-confidence.

What she was talking about was seeing with new eyes—a shift in perspective. When I was diagnosed with breast cancer, it was those new eyes for inner discovery that I was going to need most. And what I needed to discover was a new way of looking at what was happening to me.

The good news is, how you look at what is happening to you boils down to a choice.

Before breast cancer came into my life, I was a master at stoking happiness and already pretty good at turning lemons into lemonade. If I wasn't happy, I was usually able to worm my way out of the funk by any number of tactics: practicing gratitude, working on a project, riding out the storm. Most days were good days. When I arrived at the breast cancer imaging center for a routine mammogram, everything was fine as far as I was concerned. Nothing hurt, nothing was lumpy or bumpy, nothing felt wrong. It was a typical, sunny, la-dee-dah day.

But the tech saw something suspicious. I wasn't too alarmed. It had happened before, and I thought it was probably just another cyst. But the sonogram showed that the dark spot on the film was a solid mass, not a cyst. Ouch! That was cause for concern. Next stop, biopsy. Then the shocking news. I had a tumor, and it was positive. Tumor? Positive? Now that was an oxymoron if ever I'd heard one.

I was in a free fall, a kind of Alice in Wonderland moment, where I felt like I was falling down a fun house rabbit hole. There went my typical, sunny, la-dee-dah day. I was frightened, nervous, and living in the Disoriented States of America. I was having trouble registering what the doctors were telling me, and I was not a happy princess camper. My crystal carriage had turned into a petrified pumpkin.

I invited myself to a well-deserved wallow at my exclusive, VIP palace pop-up pity party. But I soon realized I was not going to survive if I stayed in a negative mental space. At some point, I came to the following decision: Regardless of my prognosis, which I did not yet know, I was not going to let my mental state go down with the ship. I needed to find a way to keep the happiness flag unfurled and flying. But how? The whole experience seemed surreal. I felt lost and unhappy, and that was not me.

I'm not saying you don't have a right to wallow. The question is, do you have a desire to stay there, or do you have a desire to try to find a new way of looking at your circumstances that *empowers* you to experience a happy life, in spite of everything that is happening?

The good news is, how you look at what is happening to you boils down to a choice. Plain and simple. Because the truth is, the glass is half full *and* the glass is half empty. Let me back up the royal bus and emphasize that. Half empty and half full. They're both true. But if you choose to look at the glass half empty, whatcha gonna do with that? We must learn to choose to see the glass half full. It's like crossing the street to get away from the chilly shadows. Look both ways, see both ways, and then choose to cross over to the sunny side. You know the shadowy side still exists, but by shifting over to the sunny side, the shadows are no longer your problem.

My journey to find how to beat the breast cancer blues did indeed require a continual shift in how I looked at my circumstances so I could see what was happening in new, more positive ways. That I found my way certainly does feel like a miracle. That I can possibly help you and others with my treasure compounds the miracle. It is a miracle that cradles my smile, lights my days, and helps me wake up with a big bundle of gratitude in my heart—"in spite of" gratitude, the best flavor there is.

So what were some of the challenges for which I needed those new eyes and a shift in perspective when I was diagnosed with breast cancer? First, there were the run-of-the-mill, garden-variety emotions of fear and turmoil. Then came the onslaught of specific fears: the issue of survival statistics on breast cancer after it had traveled to the lymph nodes; how to tell my kids; worry over my kids' worry; worry over my husband Howie's worry; fear of physical pain; fear of sadness;

fear of being abandoned by the world for being sick; fear of facing chemo; fear of the fallout that can result from chemo (pardon the pun) such as baldness and nausea; fear of the mastectomy; fear of being maimed; fear of looking ugly; fear of radiation; and even the fear of getting tattooed. That's just to name a few.

My dad told me a Yiddish tale about troubles and worries. In it, some villagers complain about their problems, day in and day out. Finally, they turn to the rabbi for help. The rabbi has a solution. He tells them they can take all their troubles and worries and throw them on the wall surrounding the village. If they want someone else's worries, they can take them instead. When the villagers throw their troubles and worries on the wall

I didn't have to know right away how to climb out of the moat. I just needed to take a first step.

and see everyone else's troubles and worries, they all decide to take their own back. On the day I found out I had breast cancer, I had the distinct notion that I might have actually gone through with a trade.

Here's what I understood from the get-go: I knew I had some decisions to make. Was I going to sink, or was I going to swim? I wanted to swim! But how? How to swim when all the muck, seaweed, and seawall of fear were swirling around my ankles like an octopus, its many tentacles ready to grab me and pull me under.

Then I remembered something that life had taught me. You don't have to know how you are going to reach a goal before you start working toward that goal. The fear of not knowing the path, the how-to-get-there map to a dream or a goal, keeps many people from even starting. But just like climbing a mountain, you don't know exactly how you are going to get to the top. If you step where you can see, you'll see the next step after that and will keep reaching higher levels with every step you take, trusting that the next step will appear.

That's when I connected the dots. This was the same thing. It wasn't a dream I was pursuing, but it was a worthy goal: personal happiness. My fear was overwhelming me, and I was having trouble thinking, let alone solving big issues. I realized I didn't have to see how I was going to get out of the funk and climb out of the alligator-infested moat. Here was the key: I didn't have to know right away how to swim in those rough waters. I didn't have to know how to climb out of the moat. I just needed to take a first step. And I knew that after making the decision that I wanted to climb out of the moat, the first step up the ladder to safety was learning how to see with new eyes!

The Power of Sustained Thinking

So how was I going to learn to see with new eyes? The great French philosopher Voltaire said, "No problem can withstand the assault of sustained thinking." If no problem could sustain the assault of sustained thinking, then I was going to wage an assault the likes of which Attila the Hun himself had never seen.

Imagine you're in the ocean. There's a powerful riptide, and you can't swim to shore. Your task right now is not to try to swim to shore. Your task is to keep swimming parallel to shore until you find an area where the tides no longer grip you, and then you can swim back to the beach. You're not supposed to focus on swimming straight back to the beach in a monster current because you can't. That's just the nature of the beast.

Similarly, after my diagnosis, my mind was gripped in a riptide of confusion and fear. I didn't have answers to my questions exactly when I needed them. What I knew I needed to do was to hang in there and let things sift while I put my mind to work with sustained thinking. I shouldn't succumb to the temptation of believing I could immediately swim straight back in to shore and have my answers. It wasn't going to be a straight line to get there. If I thought that, it would only cause huge sadness and frustration. I decided to give myself the grace of time to figure out the answers. And so must you.

I believed that ideas for finding my way would come to me over time. I had faith that if I took the first step up the mountain—which to me meant starting my thinking process on how to see with new eyes—I would begin finding the answers at some point.

It's not easy to transform fetid fear into fragrant flowers. Just understand that in this breast cancer game, mental survival can be just as much a part of the survival journey as physical survival. You've got to fight for your happiness mojo! You might not know it now, but like the cow poop that became a cow "pie" and the caterpillar that morphed into a butterfly, you stand at the precipice of fundamentally awesome transformation!

Sustained thinking does not mean thinking about something all day long. That would have driven me crazy.

I asked myself, "How do I handle this diagnosis and not lose my joy?" Then I let go and let the question sift down into my subconscious mind. This is probably what the conventional wisdom to sleep on it accomplishes. I trusted that the answer would come to me in due time. I trusted that my subconscious mind would be running the question like a silent 1920s' movie in the background, and when the answers were ready, they would bubble up from a deep, inner wellspring to greet my conscious mind. And they did. Helloooo, princess. Have I got answers for you! And I'm excited to share what I discovered.

Here's an initial peek into the first answer that unfolded after my sustained thinking spree. I will get into depth on it later, but for now, here is what I heard when I asked myself that question about handling the diagnosis while retaining my joy and added a second question about where to put my mind to get through it all. After a few days, an answer came to me in a very quiet way. In that still, small voice deep inside, I heard the following words: If I let cancer steal my joy, then I will have died while I'm still alive.

"Say what," I muttered. "Say that again. I think I'm on to something." I heard it again: *If I let cancer steal my joy, then I will have died while I'm still alive.*

Eureka! That was it! That was the shift in perspective that my sustained thinking, my asking myself a good question, brought me to. I replayed that answer inside my mind over and over during my cancer journey when I got off course and started falling into sadness. It reminded me that I had a choice. I could let cancer steal my joy, but as I like to say, what was I gonna do with that? Did I want to live the rest of my allotted life in a state of misery? I might as well hang up my toe shoes and walk home without my tutu. I chose *nyet* to that option. Instead, I chose no *theft* for whatever time I had left. I chose happiness.

Look for ways to take a positive approach to how you perceive what is happening to you.

Now all I needed were the strategies, the how-to stuff to lead me to that promised land of happiness. That's where the buried treasure lies, and that is what I am happily sharing with you.

Lest you think that I am Princess Zen Master—all calm and able to figure things out easily—and that every dip into my inner-well-spring-wisdom produces perfectly profound answers, my reply would be, "Fat chance. From your mouth to God's ears." Here's some insight. When I was born, I was covered with a rash from head to toe. Why? The doctor said I had a Cadillac motor in a Ford chassis. I'm not high-strung, and I'm not a drama mama, but I do tend to be a nervous Nellie. I worry, not to the point of obsession, but there have been more than a few times when I have had to talk myself off the ledge with the help of a friend. There's a good chance I am not made of calmer stuff than you.

There's no dog and pony trick, no sleight of hand, when it comes to mental survival. It's a thing, and you must find the thing or combination of things that work for you. Try on the strategies and tips I offer like that fascinator you ordered for the Royal Ascot horse races. Make up your own tips and tricks. Write them down so you remember them. To the extent that I can truncate this process for you with ideas for happiness that you might not have thought of, I'll be happier than a pachyderm in a no-poach zone.

Nobody gets through life without some bumps, scrapes, scratches, and stuff that literally almost kills us. And here's a newsflash from my bailiwick's bulletin: In the end, something always kills us.

Take your first step out of the alligator-infested moat by deciding you want to see with new eyes. Then look for ways to take a positive approach to how you perceive what is happening to you. And if you were never that happy before, it's not too late to set your sails in that direction. Maybe now is your time. Maybe that's your angle to see this breast cancer thing as a gift. Maybe this is your blessing in disguise. For me, there was a palace pant load of blessings in disguise.

Having the honor and good feeling of helping you is just one of them.

If I let cancer steal my joy, then I will have died while I'm still alive.

2

An Optimistic Perspective

Optimism is optimizing your chances for a better outcome.
–Princess Diane von Brainisfried

S o what happened next, after I gave myself the grace of time to learn how to see with new eyes? I decided I was going to look in all the nooks and crannies of my days and nights for shifts in perspective to translate what was happening in a positive and optimistic manner. I started by keeping my eyeballs peeled like a banana in Jane Goodall's goodie bag. Making these shifts is a key talent of optimists. It's also called reframing, and it's a key skill for becoming happier.

For example, just when you think you've really stepped in it and you're cursing your shoe, the field, and the cow that pooped in the field, you look up and see a beautiful vista of lilies, heather, and buttercups. You realize that the very thing you have been cursing is really an instrument of glorious transformation. You've learned the art of seeing with new eyes.

Here's a rather funny example of how seeing with new eyes helped me handle some of the slings and arrows of breast cancer. For most of my life, my hair frizzed very easily, and I wasn't fond of that. I didn't feel good about myself when my hair was frizzy. I felt less feminine, and I felt I looked like crap. I also didn't like my frizzy-tending hair because it was a pain in my princess *tuchass*. In general, I put a lot of time and effort into making it smooth and straight. Yet my hair was always vulnerable to freaking out. Rain, humidity, and even a spit caught in the wind put my hair at risk for a frizz. Everywhere I went, I had to carry a rain hat. I wished I didn't have that hair.

And then, poof! Be careful what you wish for. Forget the perils of feeling crappy from frizzy hair. Suddenly I had *no* hair. But something interesting happened that changed my perspective forever and gave me new eyes to see something wonderful about frizzy hair. When my bald dome started sprouting new growth after chemotherapy, I noticed it was coming in with a very different texture. Instead of thick, sturdy, frizz-able brisket hair, it came in silky and fine, and it was totally unfrizzy-able. I liked to call it "mailman hair" because neither rain nor snow could frizz it back to normal. The problem was, it wasn't me! I didn't recognize this corn silk flowing on my head. This new hair identity was symbolic of just one more item in the checkout counter of breast cancer insults and onslaughts to my identity.

Then I went outside one fine, wet, humid, disgusting, but fabulous summer day, and my new growth of hair was magically and inex-plicably no longer smooth and silky. It went *poof* and looked like crap. I was exhilarated because I was back! I loved my frizzy hair and all it symbolized. It symbolized my health returning, my authenticity, and my gratitude for even having hair at all. All it took was seeing with new eyes.

What Optimism Is

There's an old tale that aptly illustrates what optimism is. Here's my version of the story.

In the early 1800s, there were two princess sisters who wanted to see the world without having to be so princessy all the time. Their names were Princess Aye and Princess Bea. They disguised themselves as glass slipper salesmen and went to work for a glass slipper factory.

For me, beyond any impact on physical survival, optimism means psychic survival.

The owner sent them on a mission across the sea to find new markets for his bespoke glass slippers. They landed on a beautiful tropical island and were warmly greeted by the queens and princesses.

Princess Aye radioed back to the glass slipper factory owner. "Bad news, sir! Found a new market, but they don't wear glass slippers."

Princess Bea radioed back to the factory owner too. "Great news, sir! Found a new market, and they don't wear glass slippers!"

Princess Bea's eyes saw an opportunity, while Princess Aye's eyes saw a problem. The situation was the same, but they each interpreted the story differently. Was Princess Bea less of a realist than Princess Aye? No. She reframed what could have been seen as a problem into a benefit—a big optimism tactic.

Shakespeare wrote that it is only our thinking that makes things good or bad. I think he missed his calling. He would have made a darn good glass slipper merchant—although he did tackle Venice.

Martin Seligman, whom many recognize as the father of positive psychology, says his studies over the decades have shown him that one big difference between optimists and pessimists is their different ways of interpreting the bad stuff that happens to them. Seligman believes that a defining knack of an optimist is their ability to alter their negative self-talk when bad stuff happens.[1]

Many of you know the children's book *The Little Engine that Could*. That Little Engine had to have a positive inner narrative to help the long train that stalled get up the big hill. Had the Little Engine been a pessimist, he might have interpreted the situation as his fault. He might have been thinking, *I should never have volunteered for this gig. Who do I think I am? The big hills are for The Big Boys. I'm going to run out of power, and we are all going to slide back down the hill, crash, and die. And it will all be my fault for being born so stupid. I'll be the laughingstock of the bedtime story world! I'll make this one try, but if I can't do it, I'm so outta here.*

Thankfully, the Little Engine was an optimist. His inner narrative might have been, *Hey, every engine faces a few hills now and then. So what if I don't make it this time? At least I gave it the college try. Nothing bad is going to happen if I can't do this the first time. I'll just roll slowly back and try again . . . and again . . . and again.* That's why the book is called *The Little Engine that Could*, not *The Little Engine that Couldn't*.

Thus, the critical inner activity that separates a pessimist from an optimist is the garbage self-tawk when life bites the hairy moose. Since we all face bad stuff, why not learn the skills that make life roll a little easier? View negative thinking like evil dust bunnies, then make like a vacuum cleaner and suck the living daylights out of them.

Why Optimism Matters

There are so many areas of life that would improve immeasurably if pessimism would make like a tree and leaf you alone. Research shows that optimists often have a better quality of life than pessimists in so many ways, from better overall health to greater happiness and the resiliency to withstand life's travails. For example, according to Seligman, gaining skills that foster optimism can aid children in warding off depression. Optimists may have a more robust immune system and may even have a longer life-span than pessimists do.[2]

The power of optimism to inform our lives for the better, especially during life's hard times, is real and profound.

Interviews conducted with Vietnam POWs after the Viet Nam war, Special Forces instructors, and civilians who faced major trauma revealed a number of factors that contributed to the fortitude of those deemed most resilient. Among the top coping factors was optimism.[3]

It isn't a stretch to see how learning and implementing habits of thought and activity that cultivate optimism could help us face and endure the difficult times.

I don't look at optimism as being the stuff of la-la land. For me, beyond any impact on physical survival, optimism means psychic survival. I'm not talking about an optimism or hope so unfounded in reality that you relinquish good common sense. My friend Fanny spoke about hope and how it can work against you. She gave a personal example. At the start of World War II, she wouldn't have survived if she and her family just hunkered down in her home in France and hoped that the soldiers weren't going to invade. It took more than hope. Fanny taught me that having hope and optimism doesn't mean you don't take action. You take the action you need, but you also maintain optimism that it will work out. Action and faith give you a better chance. It's about optimizing your chances for a positive outcome.

I once asked Fanny if she knew she was going to survive. She said she never doubted it for a minute. She took action and was optimistic about a successful outcome.

Will fear still be privy to the conversation? Probably. For me, it reared its head from time to time. Even though I decided that cancer was not going to steal my joy, that didn't mean I wasn't going to have to stare fear down periodically. I had decided ahead of time that when the fear came, I would use one or more of my optimism tools to prevent the fear from taking me down and out.

I'd like to give you a really earthy and practical example in my life that illustrates why optimism matters. I enter a lot of screenplay and musical contests. I am about to enter another one, and boy oh boy, it's a long shot. I thought about not entering because it's a lot of work to enter for something that is a long shot. I know you know where I am going with this. If my glass were half empty, I'd probably say, "Hey, why do all this work if I'm not going to win anyway." Guess what else? I'm an optimist, and I *still* said that!

But here's the thing. I said it, and I stomped it out. I turned to the optimist in me to shoo out the pessimistic thoughts. The pessimistic thoughts would not be helpful, and they would keep me from even trying. That could really keep a good princess down! Remember what Socrates

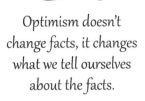

Optimism doesn't change facts, it changes what we tell ourselves about the facts.

said: "Not life, but good life, is to be chiefly valued." I want to have a good life. And that means going for my dreams!

A pessimist has to be very careful to understand that she may be seeing her life through distortions in her head like *nothing ever goes well for me or nothing works out.* That's bull crap. If you made a sunny-side-up egg this morning and didn't break the yoke, you just disproved your pessimism theory. Take that out to its logical conclusion and you'll see that *most* things go right for you. But if you carry around that bull crap distortion, then it's pretty easy to see the negative consequences that will happen in your life. Why put time and energy into something if it's just going to be metaphorically scrambled? It's really important to see with clarity that pessimism as an attitude doesn't generally serve us.

Optimism doesn't change facts, it changes what we tell ourselves about the facts. That sunny-side-up egg is corroboration for your life, to keep you from thinking that *nothing* goes right for you. You get to see through the lens of what *is* going right, a small shift in thinking with huge practical application and impact.

Each time I evaluate whether to enter a festival or contest, I have to flick away an initial inner, glass-half-empty gremlin voice that says, "Don't bother. There's too much competition. The odds are stacked against you. You're not gonna win." But then I access my inner glass-half-full-anti-pessimism guide. She remembers that I have won, many times. Never mind that I've *not* won more than I *have* won. I just need to focus on what's possible.

I recently attended the Garden State Film Festival, having won an Official Selection spot for Best Screenplay for one of my musicals. Another writer befriended me, and she told me that she has entered ninety festivals. Of those ninety, she got into twenty. Of those twenty, she's won five. What does that tell you? Winners are losers/are winners/are losers/are winners/are losers/are winner/are losers . . . *ad infinitum*! But if you live with the pessimism lens, you'll focus on the loser in you even though there's a winner in there too.

Here's the thing about optimism and how it can help with a good life. It focuses on possibilities, and that helps you take action. If my gremlin voice won, I would never enter *any* contests. I might never even try. And the not trying can make you get to Nowheresville fast.

Can you see how being an optimist or a pessimist can color your thoughts and assumptions about the world and either drag you down or push you forward? Optimistic thinking helps galvanize you to take action. When I enter a contest or festival, I realize that I might not win, but it's not a complete waste of time, because I *might* win. I focus on the *might win*.

And here's another thing. Optimism sees how preparing for whatever it is (in my case, entries, demos, summaries, and the like) makes you better at what you are doing. Each thing you do hones your skills. So it's all a win. A pessimist will just see a big trip to Timesucksville. Here's the key: Don't do that to yourself!

Bet your bottom doubloon I'm not smarter or more talented than you, but I've got just enough magic. Even so, I sometimes trip over my own magic. Even a princess can trip up and put on her pessimistic corona persona and not recognize her own magic—sometimes with funny consequences.

For example, many years ago, my niece helped me figure out how to enter my first screenplay contest online. I entered my screenplay comedy *Pyramid Scheme* in the Pocono Mountain International Film

Festival. Months later, my husband Howie listened to a phone message that said to call back the Pocono Mountain Festival. We were in the car going somewhere, and we agreed that the caller was probably trying to sell us real estate. In my mind, it was next to impossible that they could be calling me because I had won. I never called them back! But they were calling to tell me I had won and ask if I was going to attend the awards ceremony. I missed my very first red carpet ceremony!

The point is, everyone is breathing their own special brand of magic, and we can all circumvent it on occasion. Your just-enough magic and a can-do spirit are all you need. But don't talk yourself out of your magic.

It's a really good idea to cultivate optimism as a breast cancer patient. It's important to be open to considering that it's possible to survive. A person who has no hope for survival might not be as inclined to follow protocol, take medicine, be aggressive about finding solutions, and generally do what it takes to support a positive outcome—or at the very least, a longer life span.

Why We Think the Worst

No, you are not crazy. It is perfectly normal to default to negative thinking. Researchers believe we humans have programmed negative thinking through the evolutionary process for survival. Long ago, when we had to go foraging for our own caviar, if we heard a light rustle of the leaves in the breeze, our survival depended on whether our first thought was *Run for your life. I think I hear a leopard* instead of I think I hear our pizza delivery guy. In those not-so-good old days, if we put too good a spin on our circumstances, we ended up as somebody's dinner.[4] So take heart. It's not you—it's Lucy.

But now that we are no longer so low on the food chain, defaulting to negativity can work against us, especially when it comes to our well-being. The good news is that we are not constrained by a negative thinking default. We *can* join the "O" team! Optimism is really a set of skills, a way of thinking, a habit of acting and reacting.

It is important to know that we can change from a negative thinking style to a positive thinking style and then put that knowledge to good use. We can do this by adopting the skills and habits that optimists use. We can adopt the really powerful skill of seeing with new eyes and learning how to replace defeatist and negative self-talk about what is happening with positive, empowering thoughts. Make like a light switch and turn off the negative thinking!

Optimism Can Be Learned

If you've bought into the Popeye theory of "I yam what I yam" and you don't think you can become more optimistic, here's some good news. Research shows optimism can be learned and practiced, even if you are a classic, card-carrying pessimist. You just need to learn and implement new thinking skillsets that promote optimism.[5] And because optimism has been studied and researched, we know what those habits and skills are. This means that the power to change your thinking is not tethered to your DNA. It's tethered to having or acquiring positive thought strategies and skills.

If you can learn to tie your glass slippers, you can learn optimism skills. If you tend to be pessimistic and you think it's in your DNA, then change how you look at your DNA. Make it stand for Do Not Allow negative self-talk to explain what is happening to you—especially the negative self-talk when you are facing the inevitable curveballs that life lobs at us now and again.

Working on optimism skills is no different from working on any other type of skill towards a desired goal. For example, if you wanted to go from being a tennis player with a good backhand to a tennis player with a great backhand, what would you do? You would work on the skills possessed and used by tennis players who have a great backhand. You take a few months of lessons focusing on those skills. And then one day you're out there, and whoosh! You're a *reg-u-lah* pro!

Likewise, let's say the pessimist thought she was a darn good tennis player. Then one day, she loses two matches to her ninety-five-year-old Aunt Thelma who's 90 percent blind in one eye and has rheumatoid arthritis. All of a sudden, the pessimist goes all rogue with negative

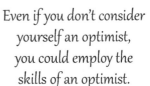

Even if you don't consider yourself an optimist, you could employ the skills of an optimist.

self-talk. She tells herself she's not such a good tennis player. She starts telling herself that maybe she doesn't have such a good backhand after all, that she's a klutz who will never play a decent game again.

But if the pessimist learned to think like an optimist, she might remember to stop the inner negative chatter about the cause of what is happening and give herself a more positive explanation for it. Maybe she just had a bad day. Maybe her Aunt Thelma isn't really ninety-five. Maybe Thelma isn't really blind, and she's taking some new miracle cream for that arthritis. The optimist might tell herself that next time, she'll whack the ball like nobody's biz. Winner winner chicken dinner. Stuff like that. She might even have the good sense to stay away from Aunt Thelma. But that could be the pessimist talking. The point is, this way of explaining what is happening can be learned and practiced, just like you can learn and practice any other skill.

If you think you're a pessimist, don't think in terms of being either a pessimist or an optimist, think in terms of acquiring skills—optimism skills. Whoosh!

There is inherently optimistic news here, princesses. Can you find the jewel? Here it is: Everyone has the power to shift on or off that switch and see with new eyes. Even if you don't consider yourself an optimist, you could employ the *skills* of an optimist. You don't have to wrangle with some pessimistic identity that you have wallowed in over the years. You don't have to chant "Every day, in every way, I'm getting better and better." That might feel disingenuous and inauthentic to you. You just have to consciously turn off the negative self-talk about a situation and replace it with something positive.

The key to learning how to become an optimist is not straight out of a Mary Poppins movie. You don't merely think lovely thoughts and then fly up into the air and start laughing. One learns to become an optimist by dropping the thought habits that promote pessimism and learning a new set of thought habits that promote optimistic thinking. Those new thought habits include seeing with new eyes, reframing, and several more we're going to talk about.

Now you say, "Princess Diane von Brainisfried, how were you able to find optimism when you didn't know whether your prognosis was good or not? After all, the cancer had metastasized into your lymph nodes."

This is how: I *decided* (there's that word again) to look at optimism in a new light. Here's what kept happening and how I made the mental leap to positivity. In the beginning of this journey of mine, in this new state of being diagnosed with cancer, things kept looking worse. First, the doctors thought what they saw was possibly just a cyst in my left breast. The sonogram proved that wrong. It was a mass. But a mass could be benign or it could be malignant. We had to do a biopsy. The mass was positive for malignancy. *Positive.* That's a darn funny word for something that seems to me pretty negative. But it looked like the tumor was really small, perhaps only a stage one tumor. So small, I was told, that it was a really good "catch" on the part of my radiologist. I was told that the tumor looked like "your garden-variety breast cancer." *Garden-variety cancer? What am I growing, a potato?*

Potato or no potato, at that point, it looked like we only needed to do a lumpectomy, not a mastectomy. Okay. I figured I had enough boob for them to take a small chunk out of it and no one would notice that anything was missing. Cool! Then there was more good news: I probably wouldn't need chemotherapy.

We did the lumpectomy. The docs couldn't seem to get the margins clear, but everyone was pretty confident that if they dove in there again to do another lumpectomy, they *could* get them clear. It was a little scarier that time because it became clear after the first lumpectomy that the cancer had already metastasized to my lymph nodes.

By that time, the consensus was that I was going to need chemo. So they decided the second lumpectomy was an opportune time to surgically plant a port in my chest to receive the intravenous chemo, which would avoid undue strain on the veins in my arms. I went in for my second surgery and came out of it with the following verdict: The margins were not cooperating. They still were not clear. The cancer was spreading, jumping from cell to cell and then hopping over cells. Sneaky stuff.

They thought that a third lumpectomy might get the job done. But reality was settling in. The tumor was larger than the docs initially thought, and it was also more aggressive. I was already at stage 2B because it had gotten into three lymph nodes. I needed chemo and radiation.

At that point, in my opinion, a mastectomy seemed to be the wisest choice from all angles. I didn't necessarily need a double mastectomy, but for me, keeping my right boob was a possible ticking time bomb. And it would have been impossible to surgically create a new left breast to match the right one because of my size.

Here's a little newsflash: Because issues we encountered kept looking worse, not better, I started losing trust that everything was going to be okay. Every new medical scenario I learned just seemed to be going downhill. First, it looked small. Then it was big. It looked like a lumpectomy would do it—twice—and then it wouldn't. It looked like I wouldn't need chemo. Then I did need it. And then I found out it had metastasized into my lymph nodes. So many shoes kept dropping, I was afraid to go into my closet! I tried to wrap my brain around it. This garden-variety cancer was turning out to have a lot of weeds.

I tried to get it straight in my mind. All said and done, we were talking mammogram, sonogram, biopsy, chest X-rays, MRI, two lumpectomy surgeries, a port in my chest, a double mastectomy, reconstruction, expanders on my chest with ports so they could be blown up to stretch my skin, four drains hanging out of me, twice (one for the main surgery and one for the implant surgery), four months of chemotherapy every other week, a bald head, no eyelashes, no eyebrows, surgery to swap out the expanders, six weeks of radiation therapy every day except weekends, and then—to the tune of "and a partridge in a pear tree"—I get me some nipple tattoos.

I started to feel like I was facing what Pee-wee Herman faced in a scene from one of Pee-wee Herman's *Big Adventure* movies. In it, Pee-wee knocked over the motorcycles of a bunch of scary-looking gang dudes and ran away. When the angry mob of bikers caught up with him, they were ready to kill him. One biker had what he viewed to be an even better idea. They would drown him, shoot him, hang him, and *then* kill him. That's what I felt was happening to me.

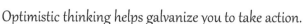

Optimistic thinking helps galvanize you to take action.

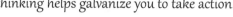

3

From Fear to Practicing Optimism

We all only have this moment.
You don't have to be certain about your future
to live a happier, better today.
–Princess Diane von Brainisfried

ear. *That* was my new reality. It was one big deal of a new reality. It was reminiscent of an old joke: Other than *that*, Mrs. Lincoln, how was the play? Other than that (my fear), how was my life? My *life*? Everything else was eclipsed by the fear. And the fear was interfering with the whole show in so far as my optimism quotient was concerned. I asked myself how I was going to be able to be optimistic with all that fear swirling around my head. But maybe having all of that fear was a good thing. Maybe it was My Big Fat Motivator. I wasn't willing to stay in fear. That's no way to live.

But the next questions seemed like Zen koans: How do I get out of the fear? How do I get to optimism when things seem to be crashing down around me?

You know, the longer I live, the more I believe that so much of our head space is a choice. We choose what we think. But choosing is not always easy. Why? Because the head and the heart don't always talk to each other. Because of that, we have to set our sails toward a decision to choose happiness, and then we have to practice, practice,

practice the habits and skills that lead us there. We have to practice the habits and skills of optimism.

Resilience is having strategies to handle whatever comes your way.

I practiced optimism by learning to change my thoughts. I practiced changing my focus. Did it take some courage to be optimistic when all hell seemed to be breaking loose? Does Captain Hook wipe with his left hand? That would be a yes. But as I've heard said, "Courage is fear that has said her prayers."

The thirteenth century Sufi poet Rumi said that our wound is where the light enters. I decided to look at optimism in a new light. I began to see optimism as divided into two camps, what I call *outcome optimism* and *outlook optimism*. I wanted a healthy dose of both. Here's why.

Outcome Optimism

I looked at *outcome optimism* in the classic way the word *optimism* is used. It is result-oriented. In other words, it's the confidence, hope, and belief that everything will come out right. For example, I was lucky enough to have a relatively good prognosis, so it wasn't a huge leap for me to have a good deal of optimism about a successful outcome to the surgery and treatment. I still was afraid, but I was able to take courage in the doctor's belief that I had a good chance to beat the thing.

But even if my future didn't look so great, I had already decided I was going to be hopeful of a full, healthy recovery because there was new medicine every day. Because of that, there was always the possibility of a miracle. I basically used the phrase outcome optimism to focus on positivity about a good outcome however I could get there, be it based in "reality," hope, a wing, or a prayer.

Outlook Optimism

I looked at another form of optimism that I wanted to cultivate and called it *outlook optimism*. I needed to make that distinction because I wasn't sure I could be optimistic if I didn't have tools to handle a bad prognosis. I thought my optimism might become a house of cards. I needed a framework for cultivating optimism either way.

Outlook optimism focused not on whether my outcome/prognosis looked good or bad but on my confidence in my ability to handle my outcome/prognosis, regardless of whether it was good or bad. To me, this distinction was a big deal. Outlook optimism encompassed the belief that I had the resilience to cope with whatever happened in the future. It also encompassed the idea that I would find a way to live the best I could right then and there, regardless of the prognosis.

My idea of outlook optimism has its roots in the resilience of the human spirit. I believe we are all wired for resilience. It's just that some of us have developed it more than others. As the philosopher Nietzsche reportedly said, "That which does not kill us makes us stronger." Except he was German, so it probably went more like, "Stronger, that which kills us not, does make us." That's an inside joke for you German speakers out there—and I'm not one of you. But as long as I'm going all international on your darn self, the Italians have this down too. *Mi arrangio.* Loosely translated, it means, "Hey, I'll be able to handle it. I've got a palace pant load of resilience." Okay, that was *very* loosely translated.

Seeing the good in life moment by moment, and no matter what, being able to take it day by day, *this* was a new angle on optimism for me. In my fearful moments, I was able to abate the fear that the treatments might not work by drawing on an outlook-optimistic worldview for strength. Whatever happens, I would and could handle it.

Resilience is having strategies to handle whatever comes your way. Each time you rebound from a shock, fear, sorrow, or any other life circumstance that feels like an assault on the palace fortifications, that's another notch on your resilience belt. Over time, you look back and you say, "Dang, I've handled a lot of stuff, and I'm still breathing! I got this! I'm really okay, and I'm going to be okay, no matter what happens." The "no matter what happens" part is a key aspect of outlook optimism.

"Well, Princess Diane von Brainisfried, it's fine that you can look back and realize you handled a lot of stuff," you say. "But how does a person handle all that stuff when it's happening without hyperventilating and passing out? For example, when you found out you were facing the bilateral mastectomy, wasn't it hard because you had a nice pair of really big boobies? How did you handle *that*? In a sense, weren't they a part of your identity? Didn't that make you sad, scared, and angry? And how did you handle it when you had to shave your head? How about when your big toenail fell off because of chemo? How about all the medical appointments you had to schedule? Add to that all the other issues besides fear. How did you cross the resilience bridge and get to the other side to do the royal wave?"

These are really good questions. Speaking of waves—granted, of another kind—have you ever seen a wave that didn't crash? No, because if it didn't crash, it wouldn't be a wave. But what does that darn wave go and do, again and again? It picks itself up, unfurls its might as a mighty wave, and crashes again. That's waves; that's life. You know what that wave is a symbol of to me? Resilience. Part of the wave's essence is the crashing property. Part of life's essence is the challenge in living that comes to everyone. What the crash is to the wave, challenges and hardships are to the individual. Every single one of us. But the waves triumph because they are resilient.

Put another way, the more I realized that I could handle the challenges and major transitions of life without breaking, the less fear I had of the future and the more optimistic I became about my future. I realized that whatever the future brought, I was strong enough to handle it. Becoming aware of my resilience was a way of saying to myself, "I've got this." *Mi arrangio.*

Here's the truth of it: Optimism is a natural outgrowth of resilience, and resilience is merely hanging in there long enough to realize you can hang in there.

Knowing that I have resilience became an important strategy for me to face the fear that came along with my cancer diagnosis. I couldn't always control what was happening, but if I could *handle* what was happening, that was a big source of comfort. Outlook optimism = princess power, baby!

Sometimes it takes another person to point out to you that you are resilient. You can't always see it in the thick of things. I realized that I had resilience when I was asked to be a facilitator at Miami's World Summit on Happiness. During a lunch break, a bunch of us facilitators planned to get our food and then sit outside and picnic in the glorious sunshine. I found a spot by a group of people sitting in a circle, and I sat down among them. I looked up and realized that sitting opposite me was someone I knew. He was also a facilitator. Neither of us knew the other was there!

He began introducing me to the others in the circle and started praising me for the way I handled my recent experience with breast cancer. Hearing his words and the way he characterized how I had handled the process gave me insight into the issue of my resilience. The way he said it opened my eyes to the strength within me that I had not seen in myself. "She had just gone through chemotherapy and radiation, and her dad had just died two months earlier," he said. "She gave an uplifting eulogy, and then, two months later, she gets up at her son's wedding—and she's bald and wearing a wig—and sings a beautiful song!"

I had never looked at it that way. At any point, I could have fallen apart. I saw myself as just doing my best, from one moment to the next—except, of course, when it didn't even feel like I was doing my

Here's the truth of it: Optimism is a natural outgrowth of resilience, and resilience is merely hanging in there long enough to realize you can hang in there.

best. Then I just hung in there like a howler monkey with no idea what to do next. If you think you're just not an optimistic person and can't handle breast cancer with optimism and resiliency, I want you to know that if you can just hang in there and get through the evolution of emotions, you will be able to step back and observe that you have more resiliency than you might be giving yourself credit for. And that will help you become outlook-optimistically optimistic about your future. It will be another tool in your gem-encrusted tool belt to combat the fear. You'll know you can take it and survive it mentally. That's mental grit, and mental grit is a powerful princess tool for combatting fear.

For me, outlook optimism is not about my chances for survival. It has more to do with awakening and acknowledging my resilience and courage to thrive in whatever time I have left alive. It's an optimism that every day I'm alive is going to be well lived in gratitude. It is the optimism that I'm going to have a life of heightened experiences and sensibilities because I'm fully aware on a visceral level of how precious it is. And no matter what, as long as I have today, I have hope for another today. And what is life but a string of todays? There are new discoveries in medicine being made every day, and that is always a cause for hope. Never lose hope because every day holds the possibility of miracles, big and small.

The outlook optimism epiphany was a pivotal moment in my healing and happiness journey. As I mentioned, I realized that for the sake of my happiness, I needed to make the decision to live—not die—in the time I had left alive. That's a really important threshold decision. Do not take that moment lightly. That's the G-spot of breast cancer—the part where cancer actually becomes a *gift*. Because really, we should live like that whether we have a diagnosis or not. When you think of it, we're all terminal, or as my mother used to say, "We're all renters."

I am optimistic that I can handle what is thrown in front of me. That is a huge relief from the fear. As soon as you realize you are putting one foot in front of the other, getting out of bed in the morning to face the day, that is already a show of resilience. Add to it enjoying your day, your kids, your life, your food, your work, and all the other potentially enjoyable things in your life. That's more resilience in your resilience bank. Bankable resilience. Now go out there and continue making deposits!

The Gift of Now

It's not a stretch to guess what my big mother lode of fear was after being diagnosed with breast cancer. Of course, there was the big "Am I going to die?" fear. Then came the "Will it come back?" fear. Later, it was the "OMG! There is no test to see if I'm cured" fear. And there were a whole gaggle of secondary fears about my kids' and husband's fears. Of course, we mustn't forget the "I won't finish my earthly mission" fear, which, for me, centered around my writing projects. Then came the big "I will never get to know my future grandchildren, and they won't know me" fear. And finally, there was the "Awe shucks! I won't get to have any more fun on Earth" fear.

I don't know about you, but I have my bucket list of last foods, which I'm thinking maybe I better eat. Want to hear them? A huge—and by huge I mean *huge*—bucket of buttered movie popcorn; a nuclear-sized breadcrumb, butter, and garlic stuffed artichoke; the entire top of a crumb cake, which I assume is made with cinnamon, sugar, and butter. Notice a theme here? Besides my teeth?

Early on, I asked the doctors if, after all of my treatments, they would be able to tell if the cancer was gone. I wanted to know if they got it all. I was shocked by the answer. They weren't going to be able to tell. According to my understanding, at that point in medical knowledge, there was no test to see if I was cancer free. Time would tell. That was it.

That blew my mind. It still does. A mastectomy, a bald head for months, chemotherapy that required a hazmat suit for the purveyors, radiated to the glow point, all my estrogen blocked by drugs—and after all was said and totally done, there was no test to see if they got it all? Darn it to dingleberries!

I had to find a way to handle my brain to live with the idea that I would not (and will not) know if I'm safe. I wanted a guarantee of cure. The not knowing was really disturbing. I'm not good with cliffhangers, especially when I'm the one hanging from the cliff. And then came another epiphany. I wanted a guarantee that I would be okay. Well, hello, Princess of Positivity! Guess what? Wake up and smell the rhizomes! *Nobody's* got a guarantee! No one has any certainty—because there is no certainty. Life's not certain. No one has any guarantees they will live to the next moment, let alone the next day. We only have *now*.

As soon as I realized that, something freed up inside of me. The terror abated because I didn't feel so damaged and fragile compared to everyone else. I got my "robust" feeling back. I didn't have anything less than anyone else because no one else knew what their next day would bring either.

That shift in thinking, that new perspective, was one of the most powerful realizations of my cancer journey. That one thought had the magical ability to calm my mind and my soul. I had neither more nor less than anyone else. Any certainty we think we have is an illusion. What a gift to learn this! From the youngest, most robust Olympic athlete to the hundred-year-old woman, everyone only has today. This infused the optimism right back into my heart because my new definition of being okay was being alive in the moment. What is

real is right now. Today I am breathing.
Today I am alive. And that's all anyone can
ask for. I don't feel deprived of time because
I have no more and no less than anyone
else. I have today! I have this moment. If I'm

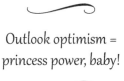

*Outlook optimism =
princess power, baby!*

out shopping for shad roe in July and I can't get any, I can't be upset
that I can't get any. The season's over, man. *Nobody's* getting any.

Lest you think I am always able to master my fears and sadness,
that is not the case. I am not perfect—contrary to what most of you
think about a princess. I struggle too, but I might be able to Houdini
out of it a little quicker than some others who don't have the magical
tool of optimism at the ready. (But if you didn't have it before, you
have it now!) I may be able to grab on to my perspective a little bit
quicker than some, or maybe I just started out with a higher sunshine
quotient. It doesn't matter. I still have my really awful moments. I don't
want you to think I don't because I don't want you to be discouraged
and think that these tools might work only for those born as optimists.
That's not the case at all.

Understanding that all anyone has is the present moment, the now,
was a critical boost to my psyche because I had the new perspective
that life is merely a series of days that I am living in right now. And
making the most of my now—stopping to smell the morning French
roast, making the most of my family ties and friendships, squeezing
the juice out of the orange of life—rendered the issue of a guarantee
practically irrelevant. Carpe diem! Or, as I like to say around the
palace, "Carpe diadem!"

Everything Teaches

In moving from fear to optimism, it is important to recognize that a
life lived well involves learning. In the School of Practical Philosophy
I learned that everything in your life can teach you something. I held

this concept near my heart throughout the entire journey of breast cancer and beyond, and I believed that this everything in front of me would accelerate my font of wisdom and understanding. When we look at breast cancer as another step on our learning curve, there is something elegant and positive in that view. Not everyone gets to learn, firsthand, what breast cancer has to teach us.

My dear royal friends, if life is truly a university, we just got accepted into Harvard! Our special motto? "Up your learning curve!"

*The longer I live, the more I believe
so much of our headspace is a choice.*

4

Suspending My Inner Cynic

Let doubt claim a corner of the desert,
but let the rest be an oasis.
–Princess Diane von Brainisfried

My heart has always told me that some great energy force exists. I just feel it. I can't explain it any other way than that. This force seems like a channel that I can connect to, some bigger energy—universal wisdom—that I can access for wisdom and guidance. I believe it is a miraculous and marvelous energy source that we are all a part of, and if we listen and feel, we can tap in to it. It is in us and swirls among us. I characterize this feeling as my spirituality.

Before I was diagnosed with breast cancer, I had a saying: Let go, be loving, and let the Divine Swirl move you. And it is that energy source, that connection to universal support of the Divine Swirl that helped sustain me through the very first steps in the new world as a breast cancer patient.

This support arrived in the form of meaningful signs, symbols, and unlikely coincidences. I'd like you to keep your mind open to the possibility that this energy exists, even if you are skeptical to the bone right now. You don't have to believe or know with ironclad certainty. I don't. I merely suspect and feel it to a greater or lesser extent from day to day. During this time period, I seemed to get bombarded with signs and symbols that the energy existed, and it was supporting me.

I'm going to share with you more about how my own breast cancer story unfurled, so you can get a glimpse of the signs and symbols I saw, how I interpreted them, and what I did to keep my mind open to the messages. I especially want to convey how helpful it was for me to entertain the possibility that what I was witnessing were messages of support from this mystical world.

The signs and symbols were so helpful to me, and they so tempered my fear, that I kept revisiting these events to soothe my soul and calm my frightened mind. Some of the signs were mind-blowing. I made a decision to suspend my cynicism and stoke my spirituality. I would let the energy do its thing, and in return, I would listen with an open mind and embrace the memo.

I'd like to show you thought processes I used to crawl out of the web that cynicism held me in because some of you will have to crack open your mind a bit—or a lot—to even entertain the idea that the universe gives us signs and symbols for support and guidance.

Spiritual Doubt Is Not an Enemy to Spirituality

I'm not going to get into a theological discourse on whether God exists. I just want to help you find a way to overcome your inner cynic so you can seriously entertain the possibility that something—some force you cannot see—is available to support you.

My innate spirituality allowed me to entertain the possibility, but I needed some help for the serious part. I found that help in the form of reasoned ammo, which I used to combat that soft-spoken cynic that lives in a small corner of my soul. This cynic is somewhat shy because I am not intrinsically a cynical person. But she is definitely there, cloaked in reason, imprisoned behind bars of pure logic. She lives there rightfully as the product of my royally reasoned background.

My parents were both medical doctors, my aunts and uncles were doctors, my sister is a doctor, and my husband and I are lawyers. We're all in the proof biz. Show me reasoned, concrete, empirical proof or hit the road.

We all have our own ideas about God. Some of us call it a Higher Power. Some of us call it Divine Energy. Some of the ways I characterize the force that I feel and plug in to are the Universal Mind, Universal Energy, Divine Mind, Life Force, or Divine Swirl.

Everyone and his jester seem to have another word for this force we intuit but cannot see. The nomenclature is irrelevant. Whatever exists, it's there for every one of us, whether we believe or not. If there's a donut in front of me, that donut exists whether I believe in it or not or whether I call it a donut or not. The only relevant question is this: Am I gonna eat it?

Am I 100 percent certain that what I feel, what I am attuned to, is really there? Not 100 percent. I have some doubt. That's the cynical part of my brain—or maybe the rational part. I don't know.

I do know that plenty of brilliant, rational people believe in some unseen, greater force. I realize that being rational does not knock this idea of a universal force out of the box. I also have no beef with doubt. My dearly departed friend Fanny used to say that doubt is the sign of an intelligent mind. My intelligent mind recently told me that God is an inner knowing, not an outer showing. I think that concept of God can comfortably accommodate the comings and goings of doubt.

Let go, be loving, and let the Divine Swirl move you.

Someone I truly respect told me not to tell you I had doubt. I am not completely sure I understand why. I think she believed that some people will be very uncomfortable with the word *doubt*. She thought I should use the word *uncertain*. But I want you to know the truth.

Doubt is a whole lot bigger than uncertainty. And I believe that it is okay to have doubt and still believe in the possibility that all this is true. Uncomfortable places make us move to what's more comfortable. What if that place helps you move more toward belief? Then maybe I've helped you. I think it's okay to use the word *doubt* because it's not something immutable. It's a more or less thing on any given day.

I will formally introduce Fanny to you now because she plays such an integral part of my life, and she is so oft mentioned in this book.

Fanny was a very special friend, the kind of friend who is also a life guide, a teacher, a mentor, and a Sherpa. The kind of friend that is family. I had known Fanny for over twenty-five years when she passed. Whenever I showed up at her door, which would usually already be open for me, she always gave me an elegant, warm greeting. With a big smile and open arms, she would say, "Madame!" Whenever I hear the word *Madame*, I think of Fanny and the warm smile and wonderful hug with which she greeted me. Oh, and of course the double air kiss.

Fanny was a Holocaust survivor from France. When the war broke out, her whole family had to hide by fleeing to the forests that surrounded her town. Fanny was a hero, literally. She performed many heroic acts at great risk to herself as a young teen during the war. She saved many children from certain death.

Fanny survived on the run from the Nazis in France, going from town to town, trying to get to neutral Switzerland. Most of the time, some kind person was instrumental in helping to save her from capture. She told me that she knew if someone was safe or dangerous by looking at their eyebrows. It was an uncanny intuition.

Fanny was bold, brave, brilliant, and beautiful until the day she passed. I know this for a fact. I was with her on the day she passed.

There was something deliriously special about Fanny, the way people gravitated to her, and if they were in trouble, the way she knew how to help them. Fanny seemed otherworldly, even though she was as real as the Velveteen Rabbit. I once said to her, "Fanny, don't think I'm crazy when I say this, and I know you are a human, but you seem to me a little *more* than human. Do you know what I mean? Like an angel on Earth or something."

I was shocked when she acknowledged that she did understand what I was talking about. "I know," she replied. Maybe angels just know. Clarence did.

In any event, I had no doubts about how special Fanny was, whether or not she was more than human. There are some things a princess just knows.

My brainiac dad made a joke about doubt during a hospital stay in his later years. One of his very best friends, a rabbi, came to visit. My dad had an incredible, quick-witted sense of humor. It was his hallmark—in addition to his hallmark brilliance and kindness—and everybody loved him for it.

When the rabbi was about to leave after visiting dad, he asked, "Would you like me to pray for you?"

With the twinkle in his eye that he had when some silliness was cooking in his brain, and with the boyish grin he had when he was about to unleash it, Dad said, "I'd rather have a good nurse."

The rabbi laughed with my dad and me. He didn't take it as a jab because he knew my dad's sense of humor. Anyway, they were basically best friends.

Dad was no atheist, but perhaps he too had his doubts. He went to services on the High Holidays, and even until the very end, he knew the Hebrew prayers by heart.

I'm beginning to think that life is one big incongruity brew and that opposites of thought can live harmoniously, side by side. Doubt can coexist with belief. It's a spectrum, a sliding scale, that from moment to moment goes up and down like mercury on an old-fashioned thermometer. We have to remember that just because we may have doubts about this support from the universe thing, it doesn't mean we have to put the kibosh on the whole idea. Let doubt claim a corner of the desert, but let the rest be an oasis.

Here's another thought: Just because we can't touch something, just because we can't see something, just because something is not concrete, doesn't make it less real. This reminds me of a story a friend told me.

When my friend's son was a young boy in a yeshiva (a religious Jewish school), he got in trouble with the principal. He was caught making and collecting on a bet in school with the other yeshiva boys, which apparently pissed off some of the parents. What was the subject of the bet? He told the boys, "I bet I can put my finger on a fart."

Of course, it's not a stretch to imagine that the other boys were cocksure he couldn't put his finger on a fart. A fart doesn't have form. You can't see it. You can't touch it. This was easy money. So they put money on the bet, and they lost. How is that possible? He pulled out a dictionary, looked up the word *fart*, and put his finger on it. Luckily, the principal had a sense of humor. Punishment and restitution consisted of the return of the boys' money and the sponsoring of a (kosher) pizza party at the school. There *is* a God!

Is there really a universal force? And if there is, can we really connect to it? We can't see it. We can't touch it. Here's how I look at it. Just like a fart, you might not be able to see it or feel it, but if you're right next to the culprit, and notwithstanding it being silent but deadly, you can't deny the circumstantial evidence. In the case of the spiritual realm, I can't deny that I *feel* it. My feeling can be likened to an intuition. Intuition is a thing, it's real, and *that's* just a feeling too. Fanny had it when she knew whether to trust someone based on their eyebrows.

Similarly, if a person is blind and the sun is shining on her face, the feeling of warmth is a pretty good argument that the sun is out. The *feeling*, the intuition that something exists, is another piece of evidence for the rational mind that a force beyond our understanding exists.

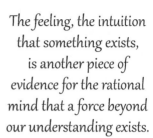

The feeling, the intuition that something exists, is another piece of evidence for the rational mind that a force beyond our understanding exists.

What I asked myself to do, and what I am asking you to consider, is to let the dial on the cynic meter lean more to the faith side. Let the temperature be a little hotter on the faith thermometer. Because I daresay, events will start happening around you that are totally magical, totally supportive, totally miracle-oriented, and you may totally miss the missive if your cynic meter is dialed too high and your mercury pooled too low. And by gosh, now is when you need this faith the most! The universe can sure come to the rescue to give you the messages, the signs, and the symbols of support that you'll need. With respect to my beloved and brilliant dad's comment, perhaps one of the signs and symbols that the universe supported him was getting a really good nurse!

Smarty-Pants Carl Jung Believed in Synchronicity

Another point that helped me to overcome my inner cynic was recalling that it was a very smart science mind, famed psychiatrist Carl Jung, who wrote about the concept of synchronicity. I first read about Jung's scarab story many moons ago in the book *The Road Less Traveled* by M. Scott Peck. Jung's story of the scarab beetle reflects his attempts to help an ultra-rational patient of his to loosen up her tendency for purely rigid, rational thought, which he felt was impeding her therapeutic process. He was hoping that something surprising would happen that would help him break through her wall of impassable intellectualization, but he had no idea what that could be.

During one therapy session, the young woman was describing a dream she had the night before. In the dream, she had been gifted a very expensive piece of jewelry, a gold scarab. While she was describing the dream, Jung heard a rap-tap tapping noise at the window. It was a scarab beetle similar to the one his patient was describing! Jung showed it to her, realizing it was the helpful sign he was hoping for, and it did indeed help unblock his patient's progress.[6]

The circumstances surrounding my choice of *The Road Less Traveled* to read was also a synchronistic event. Akin to Jung's patient, I was in need of spiritual sustenance at the time. I had been very spiritual as a young girl but had lost the gift around the time I went to law school. My hyper-focus on logical thinking hadn't helped. (Okay, I hear some of you snickering. Being a lawyer and being spiritual is not oxymoronic. I know many, many religious and/or spiritually minded lawyers.) I had been grappling with the issue for quite a while. I was longing for a way back to the embrace and substance of a rich, spiritual inner life.

One day I got an urge to read a new book from my home library. I had, and have, hundreds of books on my shelves. I had no specific book in mind, but for some reason, I was magnetized to Peck's book. I had no idea why I selected it. I pulled it out from its place on the bookshelf and read it. When I read the scarab story, it did for me what Jung was hoping it would do for his young patient.

The story of the golden scarab cracked me open. I could finally allow myself to entertain the possibility that there was more of the spiritual to the universe than I was allowing myself to believe in. It was possible to reconcile my newly trained lawyer's mind with an otherworldly, communicative realm.

Presume that Synchronicity Exists

You are, no doubt, familiar with the presumption of innocence in the American legal system. A person on trial is generally presumed to be innocent. There are exceptions to this presumption, but let's stick to how it is applied generally. In criminal law, there is another general rule in addition to the presumption of innocence: the issue of a threshold for finding someone guilty, which is guilty beyond a reasonable doubt. In civil law, the rule is somewhat different: guilty by preponderance of the evidence. The upshot is, before you throw someone's ass in jail, you better be really sure about it.

In both criminal and civil cases, a person maintains the presumption of innocence unless the applicable threshold is met. What does this have to do with synchronicity? Don't laugh. There is a thought nexus.

I decided that, just as there is a presumption of innocence in the law, I would maintain a presumption of existence that a Higher Power is real and that both the signs and symbols I experienced and my inner knowings were real. Just as with the law, unless and until proven either beyond a reasonable doubt or by the preponderance of the evidence, the presumption of existence would stand.

Having made that decision, my intuition and my miracle-mindedness were then my presumption. I shifted the presumption in my mind. Instead of wanting proof of their existence, I wanted proof that they *didn't* exist. It was a show-me-I'm-wrong approach—show me the miracle ain't a miracle. All lawyers learn in law school that it's hard to prove a negative. We learn the classic example of a wrongdoing prosecutor, with no evidence that a man was beating his wife, putting a guy on the witness stand and thundering, "When did you stop beating your wife?" That's a terrible injustice because how is the guy going to prove that he never did something?

Creating a presumption that synchronistic events do mean something of an otherworldly nature in a supportive sense frees me to live more easily in a sort of spiritual resonance. It frees me to feel the support of the universe right away without cutting down the possibilities with the lance of logic. In each individual case, if proven wrong, I'll concede. Proving the spiritual stuff wrong is hard. The cynical mind tries. But it's never solid proof, the kind that would hold up in court, the kind that's beyond the criminal law threshold.

I made the decision and the commitment to myself that I would suspend my inner cynic and stoke my inner spirit. I would be open to the miracles and messages from the universe supporting me. They would be a great source of strength in the coming days and months ahead, and I owed it to myself to strongly entertain their existence, veracity, and power. Luckily, it was hard not to. They were banging me on the head.

I don't consider myself woo-woo centric. I'm not a tree hugger. I am not a druid. I am a spiritual being wrapped in a rational blanket. I let the spiritual stuff in, but some days I don't hear the calling as loudly as others. And that's okay. What I am doing is suspending the doubt part and letting in the belief part. They live side by side, but I focus on intuition, observation, and the idea that miracles of much greater proportions happen every day.

I think the fact that miracles happen every day makes us immune to seeing them for what they really are: miracles. Miracles, such as the birth of a human from another human. I focus on the miracle of human birth, the miracle of the growth of a mighty oak tree from an acorn, and the miracle of French Bulldogs as evidence of miracles everywhere.

The inner cynic hasn't fled the coop, but my focus is more often on synchronicity, signs, symbols, and miracles. And when it comes right down to it, those things are far more befitting a princess than anything that could flee a coop.

I think the fact that miracles happen every day makes us immune to seeing them for what they really are: miracles.

5

Synchronicity and My Breast Cancer Journey

I dialed down my doubt and stoked my spirituality
to face my challenging days.
–Princess Diane von Brainisfried

I promised to tell you how all this synchronicity stuff fit into my own breast cancer journey. Here's the story. It was a gorgeous, sunny day. I was traveling on my merry way to get my yearly mammogram, only this time I had skipped a year. I'd gotten my last one in 2014, and it was now January of 2016. This particular imaging center was located about an hour and a half from my home, but it was right near my sister, the medical doctor. I liked keeping my sister in the loop about my care, which was a bit easier when the doctors where nearby.

I arrived at the center, filled out the latest forms, and sat in the waiting room. Business as usual. The receptionist called my name, and I went into the Girls Only Zone to get gowned up and ready to have my breasts pressed into pancakes for thirty seconds each. That's when my first angel appeared.

She wasn't playing a harp and she didn't wear a halo, but she was definitely my angel. Who was she in earthly life? She was the tech who said, "I'm reviewing your film from your last mammogram, and it looks like you have dense breasts. I think you should have a 3-D mammogram, not just a regular mammogram. We have one 3-D mammogram machine, and since it just happens to be free for use right now, I'm going to put you on that machine."

So here's what I was thinking: *You're kidding me? You have one 3-D machine and it just happens to be free this moment? And in your best judgement, that's the machine I should be using because of my dense breasts? And you're giving me this grace, even though I don't have a prescription for 3-D imaging? Holy shitake mushrooms. It's my lucky day!* Little did I know, synchronicity was afoot!

I sometimes wonder if things would have turned out as "well" if I had gotten another tech or if the 3-D mammography machine hadn't been free. I'm not sure. I don't know if what was picked up on the 3-D equipment also would have been picked up on a "regular" machine. I'm no princess doctor. In any case, better to be lucky than smart.

After my mammogram, my angel returned with an air of concern. The doctors had seen something on the film. The doctor wanted me to have a sonogram to see whether we were dealing with a solid mass or merely a cyst. She explained that a cyst, as opposed to a solid mass, is filled with fluid. Her description reminded me of those individually wrapped chocolate-covered cherries displayed at gas station and drugstore checkout counters. You know the kind. When you bite into them, there's a cherry inside and some sort of cherry goop that oozes out. I love those things. That's what I was thinking, in addition to the beginning rumblings of volcanic panic. Just the very first embers.

I was talking to myself to keep calm. I reminded myself of my previous do-over mammograms, although I'd never needed a sonogram. The chocolate-covered cherry stuff seemed a tad more serious. But still, I wasn't pushing the big red panic button. Not yet. They often saw stuff they were unsure of. It was just my large, dense, cystic breasts giving them a run for their money. A big-bosomed gal had to take

the good with the bad, after all. It was
probably just a cyst. I'd had sonograms
when I was pregnant to make sure the
baby was coming along great. So maybe
this was the same thing. They just wanted
to make sure my breasts were coming along great. That was it.

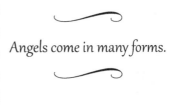

Angels come in many forms.

Besides, the idea of having breast cancer was just too far out. Breast cancer was over *there*—and I was over *here*. This was not within Princess Diane von Brainisfried's vicinage. This kind of thing, the Big C, was in the backyard of someone else's kingdom. Everything was still okay. Everything was still normal. I was joking and laughing as usual. Strangers were smiling at me.

They took me to a dark room and did the sonogram. Warm jelly, cold wand. I listened to the whir and thump of the machine and watched the tech's face as she listened to the whir and thump of the machine. I watched her expression the way I watched a flight attendant's face during jet turbulence. I looked for signs of distress: a slight furrowing between the eyes, tightness, a concerned look. And I was pretty sure that I saw them. She didn't like what she was seeing, and I didn't like what I saw when she was seeing it.

There was a shift of energy, a shift in my heart and in my mind. Fear was creeping in. Fear changed everything, as it always does. I tried to handle the fear. I told myself to take a closer look at it. What was it really? It couldn't be touched or seen. When told to face my fear, I could not really do that because it was nowhere. I decided that fear didn't really exist except in the dictionary, that it only had fangs if I let it, that it was a big bag of wind. I couldn't put my finger on it, just like that fart. But just like that fart, it could be smelled.

The nurse came back. The verdict was in. This was no chocolate-covered cherry with liqueur in the middle. I did not have a cyst. This was a solid mass. I was going to need a biopsy. The pit of my stomach was in knots. I was scared, and it all felt surreal. My world was suddenly upside down, and it felt as if I were having an out-of-body experience. This couldn't be happening to me.

I knew, theoretically, that those feelings would pass, but I was pure jellyfish-no-brain-emotion and numbness at the same time. No area of my brain was mobilizing to grab my attention and find some stabilizing emotion. I was in free fall mode.

And yet, I had been practicing positive psychology principles for a long time. Running in the back of my mind like the subtitles in a foreign movie was the belief that I would find my way to more solid ground at some point. I would do this, not because I was some sort of superhero princess, but because I was superhumanly uncomfortable in that place of fear. I knew instinctively that I had to figure out some other place for my head to reside. But I was on unfamiliar emotional turf. I usually felt safe in the world. That day, feeling safe was a faraway harbor.

They say there are no atheists in foxholes. The foxhole cameth.

When I got through the sonogram and the shock of there being something on the sonogram screen worth worrying about, the nurses asked if I wanted them to do the biopsy right then and there. In one sense, that was fantastic because I wouldn't be kept in suspense any longer than necessary. But I was afraid, and I wanted to know if it hurt. The answer was insanely unhelpful, although that wasn't the nurse's fault. She told me one woman said it was the most painful thing that ever happened to her, and another woman said it was nothing.

How could I evaluate *that*? My mind quickly retrieved the most painful thing that had ever happened to me: the birth of my first son. My doctors and I had planned to use pain medication, but after a few hours in labor, some complications made neither drugs nor an epidural possible. I was in so much pain that I dared not scream because I knew that once I went over the edge of screaming, I would never be able to pull myself back. My Lamaze coach was there for a while. She later told me that my labor was the most painful birth she had ever witnessed. I was fifteen hours in labor, most of the time on a Pitocin drip that was supposed to accelerate the process and increase the strength of the contractions. I had wave upon wave of crashing, excruciating, relentless contractions for hours and hours, but I never dilated past four centimeters.

Mercifully, they put me out of my pain with an emergency C-section, bumping a woman about to have triplets. I later found out that the C-section was done not out of mercy but because my innocent little unborn boy was shooting meconium out of his derriere, which signaled he was in fetal distress. He wasn't the only one! I was so grateful to that little guy for saving me by moving me out of my misery and getting me under the knife. Suffice it to say, the pain was *baaaad. That* was the worst pain I had ever experienced in my life.

Armed with that firsthand knowledge of what the worst pain could mean, the only conclusion I could make was that if this biopsy pain was the worst pain someone else had ever experienced, who was going to save me this time? I was in full-blown volcanic eruption panic mode—first from the diagnosis, and then compounded by my fear of pain from the upcoming biopsy. I was in Philly, one and a half hours away from my home and my Howie. The clouds were starting to darken.

It was time to get some input from the doctors in my family. Besides the issue of the alleged pain, I wanted to know the pros and cons of getting the biopsy right then and there and at that particular institution. Dementia had already zonked in on my beautiful physician mom, so asking her was a no-go. And I didn't want to worry my physician dad who was dealing with his own physical *mishegas.* That left my physician sister. Tag, she was it. But my sister was on a much-needed vacation in Colorado. The universe works in the most mysterious ways.

My sister and I have a fabulous relationship, and I knew I could have called her even though she was on vacay. But I felt I was being a big fat baby, calling her on her vacation merely because I was scared of the biopsy. But baby or no baby, I badly wanted to call her, not only because I was scared, but also because I wanted her medical advice on any possible diagnostic issues associated with the biopsy.

I opted not to disturb my sister on her vacation. I made the decision on my own. I would get the biopsy right away. Also, if my Howie could break away from work to travel down from Jersey to give me moral support, that would be incredibly helpful. But could he get there in time? The doctors said if Howie wanted to come down, they would wait for him. Angels are everywhere.

I called Howie, and of course, he was that kind of guy. Of course he was going to come down. By then, I was noticing that the universe had already started to do its funky town, I've-got-your-back thing with a series of incredibly mysterious and synchronistic events. First, the angel nurse had made a decision on her own to put me on the 3-D mammogram machine without a prescription from my doctor. And it was the hospital's only 3-D machine. And it had been available. But there was more. It was January 26, and that was the birthday of my angel on my shoulder, my dearly departed friend Fanny.

There was more still. Before I had gotten off the phone with Howie, he told me that my sister had called. "You should call your sister. I wasn't able to get to the phone when it rang, but I see she just called me four times in a row. You should call her. Maybe she called me because something happened to your parents."

What? Shut the front door! At the exact time I wanted to call my sister, she was calling Howie from Colorado? Four times in a row?

My sister adored Howie, but she never called him on the phone. She called me if she wanted to get in touch. Even if she had a question she thought he might be able to help her with, she always called me first. This was odd. There were no calls from my sister on my cell phone.

Worried that something might have happened to my parents, I got off the phone with Howie and immediately called my sister in Colorado to ask what she had called about. She was happy to hear from me, but she didn't know what I was talking about. She hadn't made any calls to Howie. My sister had never called Howie—not even once, let alone four times, let alone in a row.

I stepped back to look at the events with a rational lens, even though I had already been giving the possibility of synchronicity the benefit of the doubt and even though I had already decided that synchronistic events might be a sign that the universe had my back. There seemed to have been a confluence of synchronistic events. I had gotten a series of lucky breaks.

There's a song that Jews sing every year on Passover. It's called "*Dayenu*," meaning "that would have been enough." We repeat the word *Dayenu* at the end of a series of sentences confirming that when God performed one miracle after another for us on Passover, we were so grateful for each of them, and each one of the miracles alone would have been enough. I felt like that. All of those synchronistic events before the phone call, those miracles, would have been enough. And then there was the synchronistic phone business. It was incredible, but maybe the phone calls were just your garden-variety pocket dials—four of them. It sure didn't seem like that with the timing and all. And it wasn't.

Hold on to your tiara. This is big. My sister checked her phone. These were no pocket dials. There was no record of any outgoing calls to Howie at or around that time. Not four calls. Not one call. *Spettacolare!*

When Howie came down to the hospital to support me, I began realizing just how spectacular. Show and tell is always more powerful than just tell. I saw them with my own eyes. There were four incoming calls from my sister on Howie's cell phone, one after the other, at the exact time I was in distress and panic, at the exact time when I wanted to talk to her but didn't call because she was on vacation. But wait. It got even better.

I put all those signs and symbols of synchronistic support into my mental treasure chest, to be remembered and pulled out in the future when I needed them.

On Howie's cell phone log, in the upper left-hand corner area that showed four separate calls from my sister, the log did not show the name of the carrier as some recognizable or normal carrier like Verizon, T-Mobile, or Sprint. It simply read *phone company*. Phone company? Please! There's no such thing as "phone company." It was all just too much. It was all totally beyond logic. And this was what I came to understand: The universe was supporting me, but it sure could have used a better IT guy.

Dayenu.

Here's the key. I could have chalked up this string of lucky, synchronistic events as mere coincidences. I might not have noticed them at all if I had not been attuned to that sort of thing. Having noticed them, I chose to interpret them as a gift from the universe that was supporting me. But most importantly, I used those incidents to help stoke my faith and confidence that there was an energy force or some sort of universal force—God—at work that was helping me. Maybe even angels. Maybe even Fanny. Maybe all of the above.

But then I felt bad. What if it was someone else "up there" in the ether trying to help me, like my in-laws, grandparents, or someone else? At times, I did feel that my mother-in-law was looking after me. Would I be hurting her feelings if she was doing all that work behind the scenes and I was attributing it to Fanny? That could really piss off a good angel! Maybe it was a joint effort. I gave them all attribution.

I put all those signs and symbols of synchronistic support into my mental treasure chest, to be remembered and pulled out in the future when I needed them. Like times when I was really scared. I still often look back on these miraculous events to help me feel the love of the universal energy that is there for me—for all of us—if we open up to the wavelength on which it's receivable.

Why not give yourself this grace? When you observe signs and symbols that grab your attention, see them as a possibility that some guardian angel, some force, some universal energy—*something, someone*—is connecting with you. Keep your heart open to the messages. Keep your cynic at bay and your spirit stoked.

Other Synchronicities

Not long after I finished my radiation treatments, Howie and I attended a wedding in Maryland for the son of my college roomie. We had time to spare and decided to trawl a nearby mall. It was a beautiful, sparkling June day, and Howie was driving the route suggested by his GPS. On my right, I saw the mall in the distance. In the lane beside us to the left, I spotted a beautiful, elegant, silver Mercedes convertible with the top down. As the Mercedes pulled out in front of our car, I was able to read its license plate. It read "BLESSED." I was so excited! Another message for me from the universe!

I pointed it out to Howie, and he thought it was pretty cool. But then my inner cynic got a hold of my mind. *Come on. Enough of this universe talk. This license plate has nothing to do with you. The driver is expressing gratitude for her own blessings. This is not meant as a sign for you. Cut the crap.*

All this mean-spirited inner chatter hurt my feelings. If that were true, I needed to find some positive thoughts to make myself feel better. Even if it wasn't a sign meant for me, it was a really good thing. The driver had gotten a plate to express their gratitude. Howie and I turned right, and the driver with the righteous plate went straight on down the highway and out of sight.

Howie drove up the ramp and entered the mall parking lot. It was a huge complex with a number of large anchor stores and many interesting, small boutiques. The lot surrounding the stores was also huge. It looked like there were miles of parking lot. This must have been a popular mall because the macadam practically disappeared under the sea of cars. Tons and tons of cars with nary a spot to park. Luckily, after a little circling, we found a spot.

We window-shopped around the mall for a couple of hours, then took a Starbucks break in a perfect spot by the window. A few feet away was a beautiful, authentic–looking European carousel. Sipping our lattes, we watched the smiles on happy kids riding the fancy, colorful horses. We reminisced about our own kids at that age as we saw the proud looks on the faces of parents who were standing on the carousel platforms with the kiddies.

After a while, it was time to start heading back for the wedding. We walked out of the complex to the parking lot. The entire lot that had been crammed with cars was now practically empty. And our car had been virtually abandoned by all the other cars. There was only one other car, and it was parked nose-to-nose with our car. It looked like the cars were kissing. And then we had a shocking realization. The kiss was coming from a beautiful, elegant, silver Mercedes convertible with the top down. On the license plate was the word *BLESSED*.

Couldn't Hoit

There's an expression in the Talmud that says, "Every blade of grass has an angel that bends over it whispering, 'Grow, grow.'" Who's to say there aren't unseen forces and energies that support us and look out for us? Innocent until proven guilty. Here until proven not here. Our decision. Now is the time to stoke your inner spirit, not your inner cynic. Now is the time to open your heart and mind to the possibility that these mini-miracles, these signs of synchronicity, these coinkeedinks and serendipities are signs of comfort and support—celestial kisses for your earthly boo-boos.

When I talk about miracles, large and small, and suggest that the universe is supporting you, I don't mean that the universe will always make every bad thing go away. It will not always make everything better. I am talking about the fact that the universe and the miracles might help you in some way. That could mean substantive help like healing. It might mean guidance. Or it might be support in the form of helping you handle whatever life brings you.

My rational brain leads me to the understanding that it is not the place of the universe to protect me from all harm. Otherwise, why would children die? Why would bad things happen to good people? But by keeping my heart and mind open to mini-miracles, I have been able to observe that the universe is there to help me. The universe is communicating with me in the mysterious ways that it can. Its language encourages and signals the path.

My dad's father, Leo Young (my PopPop), was a Jew who escaped Russia in his teens and forever maintained a slight Russian accent. He was very outgoing and had a great sense of humor. (The apple kugel doesn't fall far from the tree!) In his later years, he had heart problems. Once, when he was a patient in St. Vincent's hospital after a heart episode, two nuns who were extremely fond of him came over and asked whether he minded if they prayed the rosary over him. Leo looked at them and said these now-famous words in our family lexicon: "Couldn't hoit!"

Those words became a code phrase between my grandfather Leo and my dad (and later between my dad and my brother) anytime they faced a challenge and were offered a possible solution that they thought would probably not—but then again, might—be productive. In the same vein, we benefit from entertaining the notion, or presumption, that miracles, signs, and symbols may be in play. Couldn't hoit.

And really, what was PopPop doing by accepting the nuns' prayers? I believe he was stoking his inner spirit and suspending his inner cynic. Why not have all the help available to him that is possible, even from other religions, even if he didn't quite believe. It was not the time for him to be so cynical that he wouldn't let in the possibilities of healing the universe was making available to him through his earthly angels.

Like PopPop Leo, I dialed down my doubt and stoked my spirituality to face my challenging days. I focused on faith. I gave myself the grace to entertain mysterious possibilities. I used my doubt, but this time, I used it to doubt my inner skeptic and suspend my inner cynic. I looked at those phone calls that never happened but happened as help coming from my angels in heaven. Because, as PopPop Leo said, "Couldn't hoit!"

Sometimes the support comes in dreams. When my dad passed away, I had a dream that was so real, it was unbelievable. I was touching my dad. I could feel the weight of the touch, and it felt like I was poking a sandbag. I was pretty sure it was a sign because in the dream, Dad was only his head. This is significant because we used to laugh that because my dad hated exercise so much and because he was so smart, a genius really, he would have been okay if he had no body at all, just his brain.

That dream came on the heels of a day that I had been asking for a sign from my dad. I had been listening to a radio program when someone mentioned the name Yitzhak, which was Dad's Hebrew name. The announcer also explained that Yitzhak means "laughter," which was a defining trait of my father. Whoever hears the name Yitzhak on the radio, let alone explaining the laughter part? Want to hear the triple threat? At around that same time, I also received a spam email . . . and it was from Dad! A spam sign from the universe? I'll take it! I'll take it!

Keep your heart open to the messages. Keep your cynic at bay and your spirit stoked.

Sometimes the support comes in the most unlikely forms. When I left my dad's hospital room the day before he died, the last thing I ever saw him do was blow me a kiss. That was his beautiful good-bye. On a day I was really missing my dad, I looked at an old black-and-white photo of him as a young Boy Scout. In the photo, he was wearing a cap. Later on, I decided to meet up with a girlfriend for an impromptu al fresco dinner at a local sidewalk café. While we perused the menu, a little boy of about five or six walked by. The boy was wearing a cap, and he reminded me of my dad in the photo. Without any warning, and for no apparent reason, the little boy looked at me, winked, and blew me a kiss. I'll take that too.

I have noticed that signs and symbols often come in a bunch, like heavenly clusters of ripe, juicy, deliciously satisfying grapes. This is very helpful because it makes it easier to believe that the signs and symbols are not your imagination. There are so many of them, it seems like something or someone is trying to grab your attention.

Here's another example. The day I was going to have my double mastectomy, my brother and sister walked me, arm in arm, through a park to the hospital. It was 6:00 a.m., and we were being escorted inside on the first floor to a large waiting room.

I noticed a guy in the room, but I didn't recognize him. A hospital escort came to get my brother, sister, and me. It was time to face the chopping block, literally. As I ascended in the elevator, I was hoping that I wouldn't freak out and start crying or screaming. I didn't, but I was afraid I might. I tried to make my mind blank about what was about to happen to me. And while it was a little melodramatic, I kept thinking about Marie Antoinette, and what it must have been like for her when she bravely made the ride to her end of days, head held high, knowing she wouldn't have to hold it high much longer because it was about to roll off her shoulders and into a bloody basket.

I thought of the strength she must have had to summon to avoid having a cosmic meltdown. She was royalty, and they were used to refined emotional containment. Yet it still had to have been truly difficult, especially since she had to leave her beloved dog Cocoa behind. I bet she was worried sick about that too. I realized that this image of Marie Antoinette may have come to me somewhat synchronistically. My grandmother on my mother's side was from Vienna, as was Marie Antoinette's family, from the Habsburg Empire. Princess Diane von Brainisfried, I have often told, is descended from the Haplessburger Empire. Close enough. I used the image of Marie Antoinette going to the guillotine to look on the bright side. At least I got to keep my head.

The rising elevator made a stop before we got to my surgery floor. The doors opened and a guy entered. I notice that he was the guy in the waiting room area downstairs. He looked at me and said, "Diane?"

I was stunned. He was someone I had met years earlier at a few seminars. I discovered that he was an anesthesiologist at my hospital. He took my hands in his and looked into my eyes, holding his gaze there. I felt an otherworldly energy beaming from his eyes to mine. Another earthly angel? Well, the energy coming out of him didn't feel earthbound. As he gazed into my eyes, all I felt was incredible empathy and love. He comforted me this way the whole ride up the elevator. He had the kindest look on his face and sent warm and loving beams of love. It felt surreal. How is it that he appeared at the exact time I needed to be comforted?

My angel/acquaintance wasn't scheduled to be my anesthesiologist that day, but he said he would stay with me as I went into surgery. He did. He said he would come back to check on me and visit me. He did.

Angels come in many forms.

⌒⌒

These signs of synchronicity, these coinkeedinks and serendipities are signs of comfort and support—celestial kisses for your earthly boo-boos.

⌒⌒

6

Stoking Inner Spirituality and Squelching the Cynic

Miracles, dahhling. Miracles are happening all around you.
–Princess Diane von Brainisfried

*I*f you are having some real trouble believing that coincidental events happening to you are synchronistic signs from the universe because your purist, rational mind has you in its clutches, you can enlist the wisdom of one of my father's physics professors at Johns Hopkins University. Dad said he was one of the most brilliant men he ever knew—and most people said that about *my dad*, so he must have been quite a guy.

This professor was both a very devout Catholic and a rigorous scientist. Dad told me that when the professor was asked how he could be so scientific and at the same time so religious, he explained that he compartmentalized religion and science. You can do the same thing. If you think your inner cynic is only listening to the science side of the universe, tell your inner cynic to shut up and shove it into the other compartment.

Here's another trick that works for me. When I start putting my cynical cap on about signs and symbols, thinking that it is all too miraculous, I focus on the perspective that, in reality, *everything* is a friggin' miracle! A ladybug is a miracle. A computer is a miracle. A pistachio is a miracle. The sunset is a miracle. The fact that there is any sun at all is a miracle. The fact that I can witness the sunset is a miracle. Birth is a miracle. Compared to all of that and all the other miracles we experience every day—like breathing—some little ole license plate sent my way with the word *BLESSED* on it seems like a cakewalk. And by the way, cake is *absolutely* a miracle.

If you need more help loosening the grip of your inner cynic, here's another idea I mentioned earlier: Just because something cannot be seen, that does not mean it does not exist. I often use this line of thinking to help me when my cynic gets loud and boorish. Time and again throughout history, science has proved the existence of something not seen. And once it became visible, it opened up new realms of knowledge. Bacteria existed, but we couldn't see it. The atom existed, but we couldn't see it. DNA existed, but we couldn't see it. We saw evidence in the form of byproducts or results, but not the thing.

In other words, the proof is not always in the visual pudding. The proof is often in the *manifestation* of the pudding: the disease manifesting from the bacteria; the energy manifesting from the atom; the brown hair, green eyes, and beautiful pearly whites manifesting from the DNA. For me, the proof of a Higher Power is in the miracle of life itself.

We can liken this to radio frequencies. Although radio frequencies cannot be seen, there's music in the room if the radio is turned on. There are radio frequencies in the air right now. Can you hear them all? No. That doesn't mean they are not there. If you were in central New Jersey right now and tuned in to WQXR station 105.9, I guarantee you would hear classical music—or another fund drive. You just need to tune in to the right frequency and you'll tune in to your station. The music is proof of the frequency. But the point is that you have to tune in! And so it is with seeing the signs, symbols, and support from the universe.

Here's one important thing to remember: We can stoke our spirituality and suspend our inner cynic in many ways. We can tune in to that unseen sound wave by reading spiritual books, mediating, watching spiritual videos, listening to podcasts, or going to seminars. And of course, there is always prayer, either by yourself or with others. Dip into the spiritual and back into the secular, into the spiritual and back into the secular, again and again. It's like a muscle. The more you exercise your faith, the stronger it gets.

I have always believed that whether a Higher Power exists is not going to depend on whether I believe in it or not. But recently I've begun wondering if there is a "portal," an "axis of access" to *feeling* the existence of the Higher Power that *does* have to do with belief. Kind of like the wardrobe was a magical portal to the forest in the land of Narnia in the book T*he Lion, the Witch, and the Wardrobe.*

I recently had an epiphany that gave me some insight into how faith might be a portal, acting as a key component to picking up on the correct mental frequency and into the frequency of intuition that helps me tune in to my Higher Power. It came in the story of the mystical, mythical island of Avalon. Avalon was completely obscured by dense mists. You couldn't find your way to Avalon because you couldn't see it. But if you believed that Avalon existed, the fog released its grip and the island appeared. Seeing Avalon encouraged the seeker to believe in things unseen because belief is the necessary portal.

Sound familiar? That's what Jung was hoping for with his skeptical, hardline, rational patient. Seeing the golden scarab tapping on his window encouraged her to open up to the possibility of things unseen. It's not "I'll believe it when I see it" but "I'll see it when I believe it." You have to be open to the mysteries.

We all have access to Avalon. We all have access to seeing and feeling the signs and symbols. Access is not the problem. We have to *activate* the access. Perhaps that activation of the access is our belief.

When you take a shower, the water behind the walls of the shower exists whether or not you believe it. You could stand there all day and ponder water, but you won't get your morning groove and your coffee perk until you proactively turn on the knob. By gosh, what happens when you turn on the faucet? Out comes a beautiful, revitalizing flow of clear liquid refreshment.

As with Avalon, the water was there all along, and you had access to it at all times, but you had to access the access. You had to create a portal to the water by turning on the faucet and activating your connection to the source of the water. You would not turn on the faucet if you didn't believe water was there. Your belief activated everything.

When I start putting my cynical cap on about signs and symbols, thinking that it is all too miraculous, I focus on the perspective that, in reality, everything is a friggin' miracle!

In the same way, I realized that God—the Higher Power, the Universal Mind, the Thinking Stuff, the Life Force, the Divine Swirl—is there whether or not I believe. For me to make my connection to this Divine Source and see the coincidences as signs and symbols, I have to find where the portal lies. I have to do something proactive by turning on my faith, my belief that it exists.

Even if that faith is mostly jiggly and wobbly, if I give just the slightest turn to that faucet, I'll have access to the flow. If you're dirty and smelly and you just have a scintilla of a suspicion that there is water behind the faucet, you're going to suspend cynicism long enough to move that faucet knob—especially if you've got a hot date and a coveted ticket to Princess von Brainisfried's annual Friends of Furry and Feathered Things ball. Motivation is everything, dahhling.

And that's my point too. The motivation comes because now, above all other times, is the time you need the support!

Once I turned on that faith, once I let in the *possibility* of connection with The Source, The Divine Flow, Higher Power, God, Angels—whatever you want to call this realm—that's truly when the magic happened. That's when I started to feel better and better about what was happening to me. That's when I had more inner knowing. That's when I sincerely felt the loving arms of the universe around me.

Get this. As I was writing this section, my girlfriend called and left a message. She said she was going to be down at the shore. Guess *where* she is going? To Avalon. Okay, Avalon, *New Jersey*. But it's Avalon, just the same.

Here's the key about stoking your inner spirit and suspending your inner cynic: Doubt is not your enemy. Remember what Fanny said: Doubt is the sign of an intelligent mind. Belief is not an all or nothing proposition. What is that biblical saying? Even the faith of a mustard seed can move mountains. When last I saw a mustard seed, it was pretty darn small.

We all have access to Avalon.

I think that if we humans were meant to "know" about spiritual realms with certainty, each of us would have come into this world with an instruction manual wrapped up in a little parchment paper and stuffed into the umbilical cord. Or a tattoo on our arses that said *Fragile.* Something. Anything! The whole darn thing is a mystery. So that's why they call it *faith* as opposed to *known*.

My point is, I don't want you to worry that you have to do a full court press to the cynical side just because you don't believe in a higher power or in synchronistic events with 100 percent certainty. Doubt is allowed. Doubt is human. Remember, no manuals. Take your doubt and put some rainbow sprinkles on it. Everything's better with rainbow sprinkles.

Just shift your thinking. Allow for possibilities. Allow yourself to be open to the possibility that these signs exist and that they are here to support you on your journey. Use your intuition to help you. Sometimes the physical feeling that comes with these synchronistic events will help you corroborate, on a gut level, that you're tuned in to the frequency of your Higher Power.

I may be sounding like the woo-woo princess of a country somewhere in the outer edges of Neverland, but I cannot stress enough how helpful it will be for you to suspend your inner cynic at this time and stoke your spirituality. I know it's not always easy, especially if you have a super-rational mind or background. It feels like the mother lode of woo-woo. But then, this stuff really happens, and you can put your finger on it.

Recently, I was driving while listening to a speaker talk about how we don't have to wait for a miracle when we can be miracles to each other. Sometimes being somebody's miracle just takes giving a hug to someone who really needs one. Lo and behold, driving past me was a car with a license plate with the word hug. The universe was sending a sign, literally.

When I finished writing about Carl Jung, his patient, and the scarab beetle, something miraculous happened. As I was getting ready to retire to my boudoir, I heard a loud rap, tap tapping. It scared the bejeezuzz out of me because I knew there was no one else in the room with me. The tapping stopped . . . started . . . stopped . . . and started. It came with a really loud whirring and buzzing sound. If it was trying to get my attention, it sure did. *Rap, tap, tap, tap, tap. Buzzz. Rap, tap, tap, tap.* What the heck could it be?

I looked all around. Nothing. Then I looked up. Lo and behold, on a skylight windowpane, I spied a huge (and I mean huge) beetle. The thing was the size and shape of an egg (or so it seemed in my fear), and it was banging incessantly against the glass pane. I have never seen a beetle like that where I live. But there she was. Doing that Jungian thang. I rest my family-crested case.

Put It Down on Paper

It's important to remember all the signs and symbols in your path so you can refer back to them to shore up your confidence and faith. There is no use in having a bag o' miracles if you can't remember them. Here's a great idea: Get a beautiful journal and keep it in a secret spot. In it, write down all the serendipitous and synchronistic events that happen to you so you can remember them and reflect back on them. It doesn't matter whether the event is large or teeny tiny. It goes in there.

For example, if you think of the words *calico cat* and then hear or see the words *calico cat*, put the experience in your journal. Don't judge whether you believe it is or is not a synchronistic event. Just be an observer. You will be amazed at what guidance is available if you actually notice the aggregate of these small events in the context of your journey. Refer to the journal when you need a little encouragement from the universe.

Miracles, dahhling. Miracles *are* happening all around you.

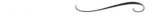

Take your doubt and put some rainbow sprinkles on it.
Everything's better with rainbow sprinkles.

7

Happiness Is a Decision

You can't legislate emotion, but you can *vote it out.*
–Princess Diane von Brainisfried

*L*et's back up the royal carriage for a second. Come back with me to the waiting room when I was about to have the biopsy. OMG! All that worry about the pain for nothing! The biopsy was practically a nonevent, a breeze. I don't know what that woman was thinking when she said it was the most painful thing she ever went through. Maybe the only thing that had ever happened to her was a hangnail. If so, it is proof positive that everyone's experience is different. I filed that thought in the back of my mind, figuring I might need to refer to it later. After the biopsy, I told the doctor she should have tried harder if she wanted to hurt me! We had a good laugh. Laughter was going to help me get through what was coming next.

We sat around for a short while, waiting to hear the results. The doctor came out to greet me, clipboard in hand, eyes squinting. Was that a hint of compassion? Did I see a touch of sadness? Uh, oh. My instincts were telling me some bad news was about to be shared. I was hoping I read that face wrong. Maybe she had eaten a big bean-filled burrito for lunch and had just passed a little gas? No such luck, *signora.*

The doctor's next words hung in the air like the drizzling smoke after a blowout fireworks display. "I'm sorry."

I'm sorry. I never thought about it before, but in the context of a doctor's office, those are two little words that you definitely *never* want to hear uttered together. My mind was racing. *I'm sorry what? I'm sorry I'm so behind in my schedule? I'm sorry we ran out of creamer for your coffee?* Fat chance. I knew what was coming. "I'm sorry. You're gonna fall down the rabbit hole just about . . . *now!*" That's what was coming.

"It's not looking good. But I can't find out how not good it is until the biopsy comes back."

I had to wait the agonizing days to find out if the tumor was benign or malignant. The doctor called when the report was ready. I heard those two little power-punching words together again. "I'm sorry." But this time, those two little words are followed by two more words you don't ever want to hear from your doctor. "It's positive."

My dear royal friends in the kingdom, before this, being positive had been a good thing. I'd created seminars on positivity. I'd created master classes on positivity. Since when did being positive become a negative thing? Since when did the word *positive* get to have the words, *I'm sorry* in front of it?

Well, Ripley. Believe it or not, sometimes positive is a bad thing. It's the eighth after the seven wonders of the ancient world, like the hanging gardens of Babylon or the great pyramids of Giza. It is in the earthly realm where positive sometimes equals negative. It is the ultimate paradox.

I was as dazed and confused as a Jimmy Hendrix revival.

Lost in the Deep Woods

What do you do when catastrophe strikes? How do you remain positive when the wind gets knocked out of your sails and you're totally blown off course—a scary, frightening, life-threatening course you have never traveled in your life?

Just as Dante put it at the beginning of *Inferno*, I was in the middle of my life and lost in the deep woods. I had no map and no guide up the mountain. I had a big fat nothing samitch. If I thought I was lost and scared the first semester of law school, I must have been smoking something. This, my dear friends, was like surfing the Big Kahuna of fear, in the middle of winter, without a wet suit. And I can't swim. Well, I actually can, but I'm making a point.

Here's what it looked like. I was sixty-one. In my mind, I still had a whole lot of life ahead of me. My father-in-law had just passed at almost 101. My parents were alive in their nineties. I still had tons I wanted to accomplish in the form of screenplays, musicals, and books to be written, songs to be sung, and good times. I wanted more dinners, trips, and celebrations. I imagined unborn grandchildren to cuddle, spoil, and love. I looked forward to holidays. I expected to savor everyday life: the smell of moist, spring earth; the sweet, fluted music of morning birds; the smell of French roast coffee in the morning; spring gardens full of white phlox and purple periwinkles; dandelions; my new kitchen, not yet done, where I had dreams of happiness, sitting around the island, enjoying wine and cooking with Howie, the kids, future grandchildren, and wonderful friends. I felt I was in the prime of my life, full of energy, ideas, and love. I felt I had so much to say and share with the world. And I felt physically great—no aches and pains to slow me down.

But now I was staring down an abyss. I didn't know what the treatment was going to be. I didn't know my prognosis. I was facing chemo, a double mastectomy, radiation, baldness, and possible death. It didn't seem like there was much time for celebration.

So, what was a princess like me supposed to do? A princess is not supposed to fall apart when venturing out into the potentially scary, potentially painful unknown.

I thought about the oft-given royal admonition to have a stiff upper lip, keep calm, and carry on. But that was not going to cut it for me. I needed a massive trunk full of wisdom to pull out when the bedtime bad-dream dragons needed slaying. I needed pithy, pocket-sized wisdom for the rain. I needed words to keep it steady as she goes. Words that save lives. I needed "Stop, drop, and roll" words. It was *my* fire, after all. But I had no words, and I knew I had to find them to put out the flames.

My mind was a jumble of thoughts after my incredibly disturbing diagnosis. I knew that I would not fall into the trap of asking "Why me?" And I knew that many people considered to be gurus and thought leaders declared that the "right" question for those in my circumstances was "Why *not* me?" Did that help me in any way? Nope. Why *shouldn't* I be thinking that this all sucked for me?

I realized that I had joined the Pink Club. I thought of all the women on breast cancer commercials, all the "Think Pink" ads, the 5K runs, the 10K runs, and the telethons (or telethongs, as I thought of them). Mostly I thought about how widespread the disease was and wondered why they hadn't found a cure yet. *My turn*, I thought. *Fasten your seat belt, princess, we're in for a ride!*

And then of course, after I started processing the reality of what I was facing, the floodgate of anxiety appeared. In positive psychology circles, we often call it the "monkey mind." It is that little fuzzy critter who lives inside our brains and loves to go bananas on us with worry, fear, and rumination. I was already starting to worry about worrying! I knew that little furry critter was gonna have a field day feeding on my worry and fear.

This whole breast cancer thing hits most of us so unexpectedly. You get up one morning, brush your teeth, wash your face, get dressed, have a cup of French roast, and say ta-ta to your loved ones as you head out the door. The sky is blue and the day is clear or the sky is gray and it's raining. Spring is smiling or autumn leaves are turning. Snow sits on the pavement or the pavement sizzles. It is an ordinary get-through-the-to-do-list kind of day.

Laughter was going to help me get through what was coming next.

Then, without warning, everything changes. This could be a movie titled *The Big Before and After*. Or *The Big Chill*. (Oh, yeah, that's been done.)

Your mind begins racing with stories of people you know or have heard of, TV shows and movie accounts of breast cancer, and stories in books and magazines. The chill of death lifts the hair on the back of your neck. Your thoughts stray to the whole lotta pain and ugly involved in treatment, and then your thoughts settle on wondering if the doctors are going to be able to cure you. You wonder if you will live to finish your projects and play with your grandchildren. You wonder if anyone in the next generation will remember you.

I never knew my maternal grandfather. Sam died at forty-six. It upset me to think that I might be like Sam: unknown to future grandchildren. It was frightening. Sometimes I talked to Sam, just so he didn't feel left out of my heart. But I could neither expect nor imagine some unknown grandchild doing that for me. And I didn't want that to be the only way they *could* converse with me.

My mind was like a racehorse on LSD. As everything converged in my mind to pose a series of improbable, surreal questions I never imagined I would be asking myself, the very first of them made me laugh when I thought about it later: *Oh, my God! What's all this stress going to do to my face?* A spot-on question for a princess, right?

Thank God I had a modicum of vanity. *In vanitatum, veritas.* Vanity can be a big motivator. I had stayed out of the sun, worn sunscreen, tried to watch what I ate, plucked my eyebrows, worn makeup, kept up my mani-pedi schedule, cared for my hair, and attempted to dress fashionably. I cared about how I looked. I didn't feel happy when I looked like crappy. And I didn't want some big old disease to undo all my hard work. But I wasn't sure if I had control over that (to the extent anyone has control) any longer.

We've all seen people who have gone through a calamity and been aged by the stress of it like a fast-forward movie—people with worn-out, haggard faces and sallow complexions who are hunched over like Quasimodo. Flashing through my mind were some photos of US presidents before and after they took office. The differences were always shocking: Lincoln, Kennedy, Nixon, Reagan, Carter, the Bushes, Clinton, Obama—they all aged like a combination of time-lapse photography and that picture of Dorian Gray. If they came in with black hair and shining eyes, they left as poster children for hair color and wrinkle cream products.

That's when I realized I was really going to have to move into action and find a way to beat the monkey-mind stress factor. I knew I had to hurry up and find a solution to the stress issue, because I had already started worrying about the effects of worrying. I had better damn well learn to handle this worry and fear, or like the presidents, this stress was going to wreak havoc on my face! (Don't judge me, people.)

I needed a paradigm shift about what it meant to have breast cancer. I needed to go from victim to victor.

I was not going to survive with my mind running away with me as it was. I didn't just need to find a solution that would help me survive with my face intact and my body in as close to one piece as could be managed. I needed to find a solution that would help me survive mentally and emotionally. The stress was going to upend me in many ways if I didn't deal with it. And I had no idea where I should put my mind to handle all of the fear, worry, and stress. I was looking for one sage, pithy, or motivational thought that would serve as my anchor and shore up the floodgates of worry. I needed a mental railing to hold on to while I took my next steps.

I didn't have the answer to handling the stress factor at that time, but I focused on the task of finding it. I employed sustained thinking, more and more of it. I wanted words to soothe my mind, princess positivity I could pull out on a moment's notice to help me recalibrate. I hadn't yet found it, but I was determined to try.

As tests came in and procedures were done, things kept looking worse. It was nobody's fault. That was just how my case unfolded. As I spoke of earlier, at first, they thought it was a really small tumor, and I probably wouldn't need chemotherapy. I would probably just need one small surgery, a lumpectomy. Then I had a second lumpectomy because the tumor was bigger than they first thought, the margins weren't clear, and the cancer had metastasized into my lymph nodes. And I would definitely need chemo. Then the margins were still not clear after the second lumpectomy. The thing was more like a traveling salesperson than a tumor. It was making tracks. They had added a port to my chest for the chemo and removed nine of my lymph nodes, but it hadn't seemed to travel past three of them. I got my cancer grade. I was 2B. That was adding insult to injury. I had been almost a straight-A student my whole life. Now I was a B with cancer?

Then the other silk slipper dropped. I could have a third lumpectomy or a mastectomy. It was my choice whether to have a mastectomy, but if I didn't have one, there was a 30 percent chance of breast cancer recurrence.

How could I evaluate such danger? How could anyone? My mind went through other dangers I had evaluated in the past. For instance, I had considered whether to ride a bike with a helmet or without one. Riding a bike with a helmet was definitely safer. But riding a bike without a helmet was probably more satisfying than riding a bike with one. Not only would it be great to feel the wind blowing freely on my face, but the helmet looked really weird because it had been customized to accommodate a tiara.

I weighed the fun of the wind on my face against the possibility of smashed brains if I fell against hard concrete. The choice was a no-brainer, and please pardon the princess-pun. My decision about getting a mastectomy was made faster than a hot knife through *buttah*. Off with their heads! Yes, a double mastectomy because I feared cancer was a ticking time boob in the second breast. Also, the surgeon could not reconstruct a breast to match the size of the remaining breast. I saw myself heeling like a sailboat in the World Cup when I walked. The only heeling acceptable to me would be done by my dog, thank you.

All of this added up to a veritable Mount Everest of stress. And then I arrived at an important realization: Happiness was something I was going to have to make room for. This was no magic wand situation. If I were going to be happy, I needed to give myself *permission* to be happy. It was the Abraham Lincoln analogy about roses and thorns. He said that we could complain about rose bushes having thorns or rejoice because thorns had roses. I could complain about having a life-threatening disease or I could rejoice that I was still alive. I knew it wouldn't be easy. I had to explore strategies to help foster happiness under these difficult circumstances.

I was going to have to *decide* to be happy. Fortunately, I'd done it before.

Tapping in to My Fifteen-Year-Old Self

Although I was a positive person by nature, I wasn't *always* in a positive state of mind. One particularly difficult time in my life was around the fifteen-year mark. I was one unhappy hot mess. I was sick for a long time with mononucleosis, which kept me out school for weeks. I kept returning to school and then relapsing. I dressed like a slob. It was kind of the fashion, but a slob by any other name is a slob. I studied, but not up to my best princess potential. I didn't feel powerful. I didn't feel centered. I was obsessed and frightened by the notion of death. I felt lost and was blowing in the wind, and I didn't know how to pull myself out of my funk.

I also had the malady we now refer to as FOMO: fear of missing out. I felt that there was a party out there somewhere where life was sparkling, fun, and exciting. But I hadn't simply lost the invitation to the party, I hadn't been invited. It felt like a piece of something was missing in me. It was out there, somewhere. I felt a big void, and I just wasn't happy.

But one afternoon during the summer when I was fifteen, I had an epiphany that changed everything. I shed the shadows and came into the light. It was a gorgeous, sunny August day. I was in summer camp on a fifteen-mile hike through farms and fields. The terrain was beautifully earthy and green, and we passed happy little brooks bordered by elegant orange tiger lilies.

Of all my wonderful and soulful campmates, I fell into walking two-by-two with one friend. We ended up hiking together the whole journey. We talked about our futures, our dreams, and goals. We talked about wanting to be more and do more. We talked about wanting to be happy and to have positive energy—not just for our own sake, but also to make a positive difference in the world. That conversation was absolutely transformational.

I made a decision that very afternoon. I was done being a one-woman advertisement for happy pills. For that matter, I was done with that mental space. I was going to make a change. I was going to do what it took to be positive and happy. I would approach the world with energy, excitement, enthusiasm, and an expectation for a successful future. I was going to get my *me* back!

As I recalled that shift in myself, that positive change I'd made at fifteen, I asked myself what I had done to make that shift. I needed the wisdom of my fifteen-year-old self as I faced breast cancer. Then I remembered: I could change everything if I just made a decision to change! When I was fifteen, I had *made a decision* to be happy.

I decided to rally that young girl's spirit and make a decision in support of my mental and emotional survival. This time, I needed to rally my mind not just for my mental and emotional survival, but also for my physical survival. I didn't want to be blue. I wasn't going to give in to depression or sadness because I knew that I could exercise my power of choice. I had made a decision to choose happiness.

But *how* could I shift my mind? *How* could I see things differently? This was breast cancer, for God's sake, not a teenager's hormone-fueled funk. I was scared. I was facing radical surgery, chemotherapy, and radiation. I was going to be bald as Humpty Dumpty. Worse, I could die. I needed a fairy godmother.

Guess what I realized? She was right there inside of me, just as she is inside of you and everyone else. We just have to listen. And we just have to give a *shift*. I remembered what I had learned and forgotten so many years earlier on that hike. I remembered that happiness is a choice. Right then and there, I made a decision to be happy.

As soon as I made that decision, I felt released from the grip of fear. It was as if a physical burden had lifted off me, and I felt my happiness ooze back into me. I decided to look upon the ordeal of breast cancer as a new and positive adventure in my life. What secrets were there waiting for me to learn? How could I use them to improve myself and help others? What new ways of health and wellness would I learn? Maybe I would even learn a few new beauty secrets. What new friends would I make? Things were beginning to look better to me.

Here's another key: One of the most important and powerful actions to take when you want to make a change is to make a decision. A decision can be made in an instant, and that instant can change your life for the better, forever.

I would choose to shift my sadness paradigm about cancer and cancer patients. I had to give myself permission to be happy in spite of the cancer.

Don't worry about knowing the "how to" of implementing the decision. The "how to" may take some searching and figuring out. It may take learning some new habits. The implementation of those new habits might take some time and practice. They don't have the expression "force of habit" for nothing. Doing something a certain way or thinking a certain way has a force to it. Because of that, you'll need to be patient as you work to uproot and reboot. When you practice the new way of thinking for a while, it too will have a force of habit behind it, one that will then work in your favor.

Don't worry about your "how to" right away after you've made the decision to be happy. The first step is to make the decision, princess! Don't expect everything to fall into place overnight. It didn't for me, epiphany or no epiphany.

The "How" in My Decision to Be Happy

Sometimes the head and the heart just didn't connect. My head was telling me a lot of rational stuff about choosing to be happy. Sometimes I could do it, and sometimes I couldn't. Sometimes I continued to struggle. Sometimes I felt disoriented. But why? What was different from that decision to be happy I made at fifteen and the other times I was able to shift my mental state and choose happiness? Nothing was different. I knew happiness was a choice, I wanted to choose happiness, and I was motivated to choose happiness. But I still hadn't found my princess positivity groove under these new, frightening, life-threatening circumstances.

During this process, I realized I had to give myself a break. In my happiness seminars, I always taught that forgiveness is a big deal in terms of your happiness quotient. There were tricks of the trade strategies I could fall back on to exercise my forgiveness muscles. One of the most powerful ones was this: They are doing the best that they can. That helped me forgive and made my insides feel lighter. I applied that thinking to myself. *I'm doing the best that I can.*

By applying that thought to myself, I gave myself some breathing space. Until I found a way to actualize my decision to be happy, I had to give myself permission to be sad, to mourn, to be unhappy—to have that palace pop-up pity party. Bring on the paper donkey and I would pin the tail on it! Hell, yes! I took it one step further. I had a right to be *angry* if I wanted. It didn't matter at what or who. Who knew? The universe? Myself?

It's pretty normal to point somewhere and assign blame. But the sooner we let go of that bad boy, the better off we are going to be and the faster we can get to our happy spot. Blame and anger are the no-win twins, but they make a cozy bed for bitterness to settle in like a winter cough. Part of the process of getting to happy is to work through grief. That takes time. But the cool thing is, while you're having the palace pop-up pity party, you can keep your eye on the prize, knowing that you have made the decision to be happy.

I knew I needed a new way of thinking to bridge the divide between the decision to be happy and the happiness. I needed the activating yeast to make the bread dough of my happiness rise. Maybe I just needed some time to decompress. But I didn't want to wait. I felt that the answer was somewhere inside of me if I could just make like a Girl Scout and think s'mores.

So I did s'more sustained thinking. I put the question to my mind a few times throughout the day and then let go. I let things shift. I trusted that the answer would come in due time. I trusted the universe to support my quest. And then it came to me. The missing ingredient was what had to come after my decision to be happy. I needed a paradigm shift about what it meant to have breast cancer. I needed to go from victim to victor.

You see, no one I knew with breast cancer had told me that they had been happy throughout the process or that it was even okay to be happy. There might have been some, but I had no paradigm for that. I had a paradigm for fifteen-year-old girls being happy, but not cancer patients. That's what was different. And I personally knew women who had died from breast cancer. Some of them were really good friends of my mom and our family. Some of them were my friends and teachers.

One of those teachers never showed me her sorrow. She was pretty cheerful, and we still had lots of laughs during our lessons. She was a hero. But I had no idea what had been going on in her head when the lessons were over. I once took her to chemo, and I gave her a colorful scarf for her head when her hair fell out. She seemed to wear that scarf all the time. Maybe she was as attached to me as I was to her. We never talked about happiness and mental survival. After her first bout with breast cancer, it returned, and she had to go through the whole ordeal again. I didn't know how she fared when she wasn't teaching the students she so adored.

Toward the end of her days, she had a recurrent dream that she was wearing white and was high above us, looking down. And then she was going through a tunnel. She kept asking me to interpret her dream, but I didn't know. Perhaps she was trying to prepare me. I think she knew what it meant because she gave me a clue. She said that in her tradition, white is the color of mourning.

Even though my teacher never showed me sorrow, I had no role model for how to be *happy* when you've been diagnosed with breast cancer. I had no role model for how to be happy living through it. What I did have was a false paradigm for what it meant to be a cancer patient. My visual takeaway was straight out of The Mummy: death in drag parading as life, face always sad, bald head bent over the porcelain goddess, disfigured. The movies and television didn't help. The more vomit, the more viewers it seemed.

It was time for a paradigm shift. My mental image of sickness would not allow me to thrive. The only thing thriving in that mental picture was fear. I had to make room for the smiles. Surely they could live there sometimes. Maybe not all the time, but sometimes.

A memory within me bubbled up so strongly that it hit me on the noggin. One of my female professors in college had told me to be my own role model. Good idea. I decided to be my own role model! Not only would I decide to choose happiness, but I would choose to shift my sadness paradigm about cancer and cancer patients. I had to give myself permission to be happy *in spite of* the cancer.

Giving myself that permission was the turning point on my journey. I was like a little kid who wanted to stay up past her bedtime and watch a movie with the grownups. That kid might *decide* she is going to stay up late, but unless she gets *permission* from Mama Bear, she's going to be in the sack at the same old time as every other night.

It reminded me of my father's approach during the last years of his life when he was living in a medical center. He had made a conscious decision to make the best of it. When we called to see how he was doing, he would say, "If it doesn't get any worse, I won't complain about it not being any better." He said it so often, we actually engraved that on his headstone. He must have understood that we have to make the best of things, in spite of our circumstances. We have to find that "in spite of" happiness.

My father's attitude had been in stark contrast to that of many of the other elderly patients who lived there. A paradigm must have floated in their heads that held them back from making the best of things. When I visited my father, there was a rather fatalistic, cynical mindset exhibited by some of the aging gentlemen living in the facility during their dinner table banter.

One guy was complaining that the meat didn't look so appetizing, to which another one replied, "Cut it in half and disguise it."

Someone else asked what the fruit of the day was, to which another replied, "Whatever they have."

My dad's response was priceless. "I'm not looking for gustatory ecstasy. I just want some sustaining nutrition."

When a veggie burger came out that was dry, someone asked if there was anything that could help it. "Cyanide," replied one fellow diner flatly.

At that point, my dad turned to me and said, "Dee, remind him of our motto: 'It's a matter of mind over matter. I don't mind, and it don't matter.'" He got pushback from some of the men and finally said, "Make the best of it. The worst is yet to come." Everyone laughed at that.

Dad's motto when things got tough was always "This too shall pass." That day at the luncheon roundtable of old men, Dad said, "Best to get the word *frustration* out of your vocabulary. Doesn't do any good."

Sometimes we are our own worst enemies. I once heard a funny, brilliant chap say, "I don't like to think too much because when I do, I go behind enemy lines." Surely, we all feel like this at times. It's not a fun feeling—unless, of course, we find the humor in it. In truth, humor was the tool those knights of the roundtable at the medical center were using to acclimate to their situation.

After lunch, as I was having a bit of trouble maneuvering Dad's wheelchair, he said, "I know there's another way out besides the window."

That was not only hilarious at the time, it proved true for me as I faced breast cancer. My way out—or more accurately, through—was to give myself permission to be happy. But right after I asked myself what the stress of my illness was going to do to my face, I asked myself where to put my mind to weather the storm. One well-known thing my father said often was that to every life, a little rain must fall. I didn't see this as a little rain in my life, I saw it as a full-blown storm. How would I weather it?

I needed a phrase to focus on, something to hang onto to keep me going in the direction of happiness. I needed a North Star to point the way and a lodestone to keep me focused on it.

After some more sustained thinking, I found it.

⌒‿⌒

I could complain that I had a life-threatening disease or I could rejoice that I was still alive.

⌒‿⌒

8

Where *Did* I Put My Mind?

Don't die while you are still alive.
–Princess Diane von Brainisfried

I made the decision to be happy, and I gave myself permission to be happy, in spite of breast cancer. But I still had to figure out how to do that. More thinking. I dove deep.

The trick to a deep dive is to ask yourself a good question, then put it out there to the universe and "sea" what trickles back. It's kind of like posting on Craig's List for the soul. You can ask the question a few times, as a kind of tickler. The universe is busy, man. After you ask the question each time, just go on about your business and let things sift. It is incredibly important to trust that the answers will arrive in due time.

Here's the good questions I asked myself and put out to the universe: Dear God, my higher power and ultimate source of divine energy, where do I put my mind to handle my diagnosis of breast cancer? What are the words I can tell myself so I can handle the fear? What are my new eyes to see this situation differently from how I am seeing it now? I put those questions out there and waited.

Winnie The Pooh was a bear who wasn't afraid of shadows. He knew a secret. Where there's a shadow, there's gonna be light around there somewhere. You know what they say: Always trust a bear with a T-shirt and no underpants! Well, Pooh Bear was right. There was light around there somewhere, and it gave me the clarity I needed for my new eyes in the form of an epiphany a few days later. I heard, in that still small voice deep inside the following words: *If I let cancer steal my joy, then I will have died while I'm still alive.*

Eureka! And I didn't mean the vacuum cleaner. That was it! I had found the answer to my question about where to put my mind. I needed to focus on that sentence and the wisdom inherent in it. I knew that was the answer I had been praying for. I had to choose to thrive for as long as I was alive. Otherwise, I would be a dead (wo)man walking.

Royal friends in the kingdom, we *must* refuse to die while we're still alive. It's *l'chaim* (to life) all the way. Life is the most precious thing. As long as we're living, we might as well live!

This inner answer to my prayers was the magic I needed to take my next steps to happiness and release the chains of worry and fear. The thought of dying while I was still alive scared me more than the diagnosis of breast cancer. I detested the idea that if I went around all blue and down, I'd be wasting whatever precious time I might have left. My days would be a total wipeout.

Right then and there I made a decision. I call it my princess pact to put the can in cancer, maintain my happiness equilibrium and my optimism, and not let breast cancer steal my joy. I was going to *live* while I was still alive.

None of us should wait until we get a life-threatening disease to learn not to die while we're still alive. To learn, we can choose to be happy. To know that living, really living, is within our grasp. It takes a decision. That's where cancer can really be a gift. If it wakes us up, we get to have new eyes and no regret that we didn't really live when we come to our end of days.

If you think that such a decision is beyond your abilities, just reach for it and don't worry about it. My dad taught me the following quote by poet Robert Browning, which is appropriately applicable here: "A man's reach should exceed his grasp, or what's a heaven for?"

Royal friends, here is another key: You must give yourself the grace of time to let yourself feel disoriented, to tread water in that uncomfortable space until you can shift your thinking and see with new eyes. Hopefully, my ideas and the thought processes I went through will not only truncate the process for you, it will also make it easier. Nonetheless, you must give yourself the grace of time to figure these things out by applying sustained thinking to the issues with that beautiful brain of yours.

The thought of dying while I was still alive scared me more than the diagnosis of breast cancer.

The process is not a straight line. It's a serpentine road. You'll think you've gotten there, and then you will feel blue and fearful again. You will feel like you are sliding back to your old, fearful way of thinking. But with your decision to be in a better place in your head, you will bounce back faster, and this time a little farther ahead. It bears repeating what my father always used to say: This too shall pass.

Regrets

There is a truly eye-opening study that further illustrates why it's critical to advocate for your own happiness, especially if you have just been diagnosed with a potentially life-threatening disease.

Palliative care nurse and author Bronnie Ware interviewed many of her patients when they were just weeks away from dying. She wanted to know what they regretted most about their lives. She wrote about the top five regrets, and wishing they had let themselves be happier was on that list. The top five!7

Of all the regrets I read about in Ware's book, this one hit me the hardest. If someone had gotten to them, if they had just known that happiness is part decision, part skill set, part habit, they could have led an extraordinarily improved life. But reading that section also thrilled me the most because I realized that I might be able to save myself and others from this end of life regret by putting in place and sharing strategies that can make us happier, even in the face of trauma.

You have time to nip that bad boy deathbed regret in the bud—and so do I—because we're living and breathing in this moment. And that means no matter how much time we have left, we have this moment. And we can change things in this moment and every moment we have beyond it.

I do not want cancer to lump me in with the end of life patients who are full of regret and sorrow because they hadn't let themselves be happier. And neither do you! Princess pinky swear—right here, right now. I want you to raise your right pinky in the air and crook it like you were a nineteenth century English lady taking tea. Pinky swear that we aren't going to come to the end of our days and regret that we didn't let ourselves be happy. From now on, no matter what our circumstances, we are going to find a way to be happier.

Repeat after me: Happiness regrets are for weenies!

Keep Happiness Interlopers at Bay

When you give yourself permission to be happy, you must learn to construct an imaginary gate around your heart, and don't be so quick to give away the keys. Don't give others unnecessary permission to steal your hard-won equilibrium. You must learn to keep out interlopers who will try to steal your peace. Sometimes those interlopers include you! Secure that gate around your mind as if there were a member of the Queen's guard assigned to it.

For example, one of the first problems I faced that breached my mind's security was the tendency to surf the web for information about breast cancer. Of course, it can be a good thing to acquire knowledge, but many times, the information I found was as discouraging as it was unhelpful, inapplicable, or downright inaccurate. Surfing the web often left me incredibly frightened. It's kind of like watching violence on TV. It leaves you rattled and in an altered energy state.

We have to remember that each person's medical situation is unique. Even one seemingly tiny and insignificant difference in your cancer "situation" could render the information you might find online totally inapplicable to you. I don't mean you shouldn't continue educating yourself, but be aware that you also need to be careful to protect your mental health. It's a balance. I am just pointing out that the internet can really give you heartburn, in more ways than one.

A follow-up call from one of my visiting nurses (another angel) came to the rescue one day when I was particularly discouraged from a web dive. I started telling her some of the fears I was having from what I had read on the internet. She said in mock sternness, "Get off the internet right now, and go out and smell the flowers. You'll be fine!" That was some of the best advice I had thus far received.

Make a decision, like I did, that you are not going to let any diagnosis steal your joy. Remember the princess pact: No matter what the prognosis, no matter how much time we have left, if we let the disease steal our joy, then we will have died while we are still alive. Don't die while you are still alive. Decide to be happy. Don't let that be one of your top five regrets—because now we all know a little somethin' somethin' about regrets, don't we? Regrets are for weenies!

When I talk about giving myself permission to be happy, I do not mean that I walked around in a manic state of bliss. That would be weird, especially under the circumstances. I had normal ups and downs like everyone else. But the key is that I had to make a mental adjustment to see with the new eyes so I could embrace the idea that happiness was not incongruent with breast cancer.

Here's a strategy I used when I wanted to let my blues run wild for a little while. For times when it was too much for me to muster a smile, when I really wanted to let loose and be sad, I invited myself to a palace pop-up pity party, just for me. I made an actual time period, a "wallow allowance" for boo-hoo-hooing and poor me feelings.

It's only human to be sad sometimes during this episode in one's life. I gave my sadness and fear its due, but then I let it know that if the bad thoughts wanted to stay, I was going to pack my bags and get out of there. I didn't give myself permanent permission to be sad. Not on Princess Diane von Brainisfried's watch!

Miracle Shift in Perspective

Was this happiness in spite of being diagnosed with breast cancer a new way of thinking for me? Yes. Was it difficult? Sometimes. Again, I needed to learn new tricks, new ways of thinking. But I did it—and so can you.

I made up a catchphrase that I often invoked to help me be happy in spite of the cancer: difficult but not impossible. I would say it as an inner, silent chant. I think I was inspired to that thought from an old Army Corps of Engineers motto: "The difficult we do immediately. The impossible takes a little longer."

And it turns out that there may also be a connection to my own royal lineage. The French statesman Charles Alexandre de Calonne was said to have made a similar statement, much earlier. *"Madame, si c'est possible, c'est fait. Impossible? Cela sefera."* Translated, that means, "Madame, if it be possible, it is done. If impossible, it shall be done."

Those French had the right idea. Well . . . sometimes. I'm not so crazy about that Marie Antoinette head-in-the-basket thing.

When I was getting ready for bed the night before my bilateral mastectomy, I decided I needed a miracle shift in thought. I needed some new way to look at the surgery that

Make a decision, like I did, that you are not going to let any diagnosis steal your joy.

didn't involve the words *cutting, lopping off, or see ya, wouldn't want to be ya.* I needed some words or thoughts to help me walk to the gallows. I wondered what Marie Antoinette's last thoughts were as she faced the guillotine.

I thought about what I was going to face the next day. I was going into surgery as a *zaftig*, big-breasted woman, and coming out as the poster child for House of Pancakes. I would also have four, yard-long clear plastic tubes piercing through and hanging down from my armpits, which anyone with a brain could mistake for dog leashes.

I was pondering how not to let cancer steal my joy. I could do all the proselytizing in the world about choosing to be happy, but if I didn't nab that how-to, there was gonna be a lot of rain on my parade. Women had to get pretty creative to get through an experience like this. I was loathe to call it trauma because I knew that people faced worse, but it sorta, kinda felt like trauma.

All of a sudden, the miracle shift in perspective came. I remembered what I told Fanny when she knew she was facing death and asked me how she was going to get through. "Say yes to the adventure!" I had replied. And now it was my turn.

I decided to consider my breast cancer journey an adventure. And I decided to say yes to it. That one shift in thinking—seeing it as an adventure—was a workhorse of a strategy for holding happiness in my heart as I went through breast cancer and the treatment. Just that small shift in how I viewed the situation—not as an ordeal (though it was), and not as a trauma (though it was), but as an adventure (which it also was)—created a miracle of new eyes. It was uplifting. It was transformational. An adventure is something you look forward to. An adventure carries hopeful expectations. An adventure is something positive. I most certainly needed a positive angle before my ample bosom became a thing of the past.

Once I realized that I could view the breast cancer journey as an adventure and not a curse, once I made that shift in my thinking, miracles happened. My heart wasn't so heavy. Think about how different it makes you feel if you call something a trip versus a trek. One sounds fun; the other sounds like a chore. The word *adventure* and the world of adventure are packed with fun.

And that shift all started because of what I had told Fanny, years earlier. After Fanny was diagnosed with cancer, she resided in a rehab center, where I frequently visited her. Fanny had a brilliant mind, and her signature (besides her style) was her amazing wit, humor, and repartee. I believe Fanny knew she was dying, and at a certain point, she wasn't speaking or communicating very well anymore.

That's why it kind of stunned me when she asked me, "Didi, how am I going to handle this?" when I was visiting her one day.

How was I going to answer that question? How could I put Fanny's heart at ease when she just lobbed me the Big Kahuna of all life questions? I could more easily steal the Queen Mother's crown jewels than know how to answer such a question.

I was struck with the enormity of the responsibility to come up with an authentic answer that made sense, that was real. That wonderful, brilliant French woman suffered no fools. I had to figure out a way to help my dying friend. I felt a huge obligation to ease her suffering with something affirmative. I had to give advice to one of my dearest, most intelligent friends on how to get through the process of dying when she knew she was dying. I felt panic and prayed for guidance.

Guidance came to me in a thunderbolt as a miracle shift in perspective. *Tell her to think of it as an adventure!* And that is what I told her. "Fanny, think of it as an adventure."

Lo and behold, Fanny's face brightened. She mulled it over, and then she said, "*Yes!* I will say *yes* to this adventure!

When I was able to see Fanny's situation as an adventure, one that I was accompanying her on for at least part of the way, not only did I help *her*, but I helped *myself* handle her impending death. We were going on her end-of-life adventure together!

I could not have envisioned that years later, when I needed help to shift my perspective, the epiphany that I had used to help her would help me help myself. As is often the case, in giving we receive.

Everything Is a Plus

Fanny used to say, "Everything is a plus." She told me she learned that from her mother. Both of them survived the horrors of WWII, on the run from Nazis. They were in fear for their lives every single day for years, and they experienced trauma, again and again, when loved ones perished and when they bore witness to countless atrocities. That's why I took to heart their worldview that everything is a plus, and so should you. After everything they went through, and after experiencing the worst of humankind, they still believed that everything in life is a plus. And if they could, so can we!

My job was to find the plus. Saying yes to the adventure had just become my go-to strategy the night before my mastectomy. I saw it as part of the river of adventure I was flowing through. If it was what I *told* myself about what was happening that was important, not what was happening, as that yoga teacher had wisely pointed out, then I needed ways to see the upcoming surgery in a positive light. I needed to find the benefits of having a mastectomy—the pluses, as Fanny would have put it. To my surprise, there were many.

I didn't put the positives in a plus column and the downsides in a minus column. The purpose was not to weigh the pluses and minuses of having a mastectomy. That train had already left the station. It was not an exercise to decide whether to have the surgery in the first place. The purpose of the strategy was to find ways to see the mastectomy as an adventure so I could get through the surgery with mental strength. The purpose was to shore me up and keep me from freaking out. My only job was to focus on the plus.

Here are the pluses I thought of. (I bet you can think of a few or even many more. If you do, pass them on and help the next person.)

1. My large breasts made it impossible for me to find a sports bra that actually did what it was supposed to do. Running as a form of exercise was never an option, not that I wanted to run.

2. My shoulders had deep furrows where my bra straps dug in. I was worried they were going to be permanent. I thought it looked icky poo poo and wrecked otherwise nice-looking shoulders. Now my shoulders would be nice!

3. I could never wear those sexy little spaghetti strap numbers, let alone strapless frocks and romantic, delicate gowns. Totally out of the question. I needed an over-the-shoulder boulder holder AAT (At All Times). This was truly annoying, for as you know, as a princess, I go to a lot of galas and balls. It can be quite limiting if you can't wear a strapless number or at least spaghetti straps.

4. Button-down blouses were another no-go. The middle button was useless unless I bought two sizes larger than I needed, which made for a terrible fit. So the princess preppy look—fahghedaboudit.

5. There was so much boob showing when I wore those cute little low-cut, scoop-neck T-shirts with thin material that I always felt a little out of place in them, both literally and "figure-atively."

6. My brother added another positive spin. He said that practically every other woman on Park Avenue had gotten a boob job, so I was in good company. I told myself I was a Park Avenue Princess. Not a bad thing, really.

7. This could save my life. Duh.

And while I was busy living, I was going to be able to rock these new perky breasts while I went for a run wearing an athletic bra (or no bra) under a sexy T-shirt under a button-down shirt under a strapless ball gown. Unimaginable!

Make no mistake. I couldn't always muster a great attitude. Sometimes the pluses got fear-filled with pus.

This often happened when I thought about the sobering fact that I was dealing with breast cancer that had hitched a ride onto a few lymph nodes. Then I would start worrying that I might die. That's when the dancing goblins had a field day in my head. I would start spinning the catastrophe scenario. The thoughts would hit-and-run me that my life was in jeopardy. The cancer had metastasized into my lymph nodes. What if it spread? I had heard that breast cancer isn't always just breast cancer. Doctors worry that it will go someplace else. I would get the cold chills from fear thinking about the possibility that maybe the cancer would spread even more. So where did I put my mind for that?

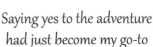

Saying yes to the adventure had just become my go-to strategy the night before my mastectomy.

Things Aren't Always as Bad as They Seem

When those freaky grappling hooks gripped me, I rallied an additional strategy that helped me a lot. I reminded myself that often, things are not as bad as they seem.

This is an extremely powerful technique to help calm down when "facts" seem to indicate that there's a big problem ahead. What we see as fact isn't always factual. And I had a string of examples from the playbook of my life that proved the point. Some were even funny.

When my son, Harry, was about four years old and Max was one, we attended a wedding about an hour and a half from our home. We hired a babysitter to watch the kids. The sitter was a mature-aged woman with a thick Hungarian accent.

The wedding took place at a fancy venue with a winding Cinderella-like staircase. During the fancy meal at the fancy venue, we received an urgent message to go to the office phone. (This was in the days before cell phones.) There had been an accident, and something had happened to Harry.

An accident? Something happened to Harry? Panic at the disco, baby! I remember running down and around, down and around, down and around the winding staircase in my (non-strapless) gown and heels. It seemed like I was in a slow-mo movie as I tried to fly to the bottom of the staircase. And the whole time I was flying, I was filled with fear, imagining all sorts of horrible scenarios.

I finally made it to the office and grabbed the phone from the office manager, who was holding it in the air. The thick black phone cord uncoiled like a cobra about to strike. I put the snake's head up to my ear, and on the other end of the line, I heard the Hungarian babysitter heaving with sobs. "Dee-anna, Dee-anna. I'm soh so-ree. I'm soh so-ree."

I was almost ready to faint. I asked her to calm down and tell me what happened. She replied, "Eeets-a Hah-ree! Hee'z-ah . . . hee'z-ah . . . hee'z-ah . . ."

At this point I was beyond frantic—beyond the beyond. I was somehow able to spit out, "He's *what*?" There seemed to be only one option, one outcome, one answer, to the impending fill-in-the-blank half-statement of this mad-libbing lady. I was thinking that she was going to say, "*Heez-ah* dead!"

But I was wrong! Thank the Lordy! Still sobbing, the babysitter spit out, "Hee'za feen-gah. Hee cut his *peen*-kee *feen*-gah."

By that time, I didn't care if the damn pinky was cut off because my little baby boy was alive! A few stiches and he would be good as new.

As I was staring down breast cancer and the fear was getting the best of me, as I was indulging in catastrophe thinking, my mind would wander back to that incident. When the call came in from the babysitter that there had been an accident, I had thought that the only possible reason for her sobbing was that something tragic—like death—had happened. And I remembered that it hadn't been tragic after all. Sometimes things weren't as bad as they seemed.

A plus had actually resulted from the incident. In an effort to comfort Harry, an ambulance crew member picked up one of Harry's favorite stuffed animals to travel with him to the hospital. That kindness shown to my little son on the part of a stranger had made a big impact on me. Like we princesses do, when I had the opportunity to pay it forward, I did.

I'm on the auxiliary board of the Robert Wood Johnson Hospital, and because of that experience, my board members and I initiated a program to which we donated beautiful, plush stuffed animals to the Robert Wood Johnson pediatric ambulance drivers to comfort the young patients they brought to the hospital.

My dad always said that sometimes, the thing that seemed the worst of luck turned out to be the best of luck. There's an ancient Taoist story that illustrates that point. My version of it goes something like this.

A Chinese farmer acquires a horse that promptly runs away. A neighbor comes by, hears about the horse, and says to the farmer, "Oy! That's bad news, man. That sucks!"

The farmer shrugs his shoulders up to his ears and replies, "Good news, bad news. Who knows?"

The horse returns to the house, and lo and behold, he has brought another horse with him. Looks like good news, right? Not so fast. The farmer's son hops on the second horse, takes him for a spin, falls off, and breaks his leg in three places. And the orthopedist is on vacation.

The neighbor comes around again and says, "So sorry for your bad news."

The farmer retorts, "You're not such a quick study, are you, buddy? Or did you not get the memo? Good news, bad news. Who knows?"

A few days later, the emperor and a bunch of his big, brawny don't-mess-with-me army brutes march through the town. Under force of arms, he takes away all the able-bodied young men from the town to fight in a war. The farmer's son, being lame from the horse ride, gets to stay in bed and watch old reruns of *Shanghai Express*. Good news, right? Yeah, if you're a Marlene Dietrich buff. If you're not, not so much.

The point of the story is that if you think something seems bad, it might not be as bad as it looks. And Fanny taught us that everything is a plus.

⌣――⌐

My dad always said that sometimes, the thing that seemed the worst of luck turned out to be the best of luck.

⌣――⌐

9

Family and Friends

Positivity will help them through, and by helping them,
you will help you.
–Princess Diane von Brainisfried

ow we come to one of the mother lode issues, how to tell family and friends. This issue was a biggie for me, as it is for many people. I was incredibly anxious about how I was going to break the news to my kids. I was also worried how I was going to tell my ninety-three-year-old dad. They have a term for people who concurrently have to care for their elderly parents and their children: the sandwich generation. This was the sandwich worry.

My wonderful, beautiful mom had dementia, so that was a blessing in disguise. I wasn't going to have to tell her. That said, a mom is always a mom. By force of intuition and the imprint of motherhood, Mom told my father, "You know, something's up with Dee, but I don't know what it is," a few months into my treatments. Wow!

I also caught a break with not having to break it to Howie because he knew everything the minute I knew. Thankfully, I didn't have to watch his face as I told him. And there were benefits in having him know everything. I found it extremely helpful to have another pair of ears listening to what the doctors said. Even though I am a lawyer, and you would think my ability to process information would be at least average or above, I found it challenging to absorb what the doctors were telling me. I found the information overwhelming because I was overwhelmed.

There are so many statistics being thrown at you—survival rates, studies, and a general overload of information—and there are so many decisions to be made. Being in a state of overwhelm is not the best state to make life-and-death decisions. It's incredibly beneficial to have a trusted person with you when you are trying to take in all the new medical information.

Furthermore, I often found that even when I was receiving positive news, if there was even one aspect of not-so-positive news, the negative news was practically the only part that registered in my brain. I found it difficult to process and evaluate what the doctors were explaining to me because the negative piece tended to cancel out all the good news. Then I was no longer able to evaluate the situation and went into I'm-going-to-die mode.

Even if the news wasn't horrible, I would take it as horrible because it was cancer, after all. I couldn't understand the nuances. Howie kept having to repeat to me anything encouraging the doctors were saying because, especially in the beginning stages of this journey, I had trouble evaluating and reconciling the information. It's incredibly important to process the information correctly so you can make prudent and wise decisions for treatment.

I don't believe there is only one right way to break it to your kids. It's not a one-size-fits-all endeavor.

Some kids may be better off with a buffer, and some might be better off hearing it from you first. Some kids might want to talk and ask questions. Others may not want to engage. Some might feel a sense of guilt at their initial thoughts. In any case, throw a little self-compassion your own way. You are not a mind reader. And hopefully, this is your first rodeo. Just do them a solid: When you or someone else breaks the news to them, make sure that the kids aren't eating their favorite food.

My goal in telling my kids was to find a way to reframe the news in a positive light. The practice and skill of finding a more positive way to look at a situation is known as reframing. I wanted to reframe the situation in a positive light not only to buffer the blow for my kids but to buffer the blow to me at having to tell my kids something that would be painful for them to hear. If I could not find something positive in the task of telling them I had breast cancer, that was going to be too painful for *me*. I had to find a positive angle. Otherwise, it would have been like watching their faces when they were very young and having to tell them that there really *were* monsters under their bed. "I saw them, they were for real, and they looked hungry. And by the way, kids, it's bedtime!"

I came upon the following idea. In breaking the news to my kids, as well as to my family and friends, I would endeavor to do three things: reframe the news in as positive a light as possible, keep the rhythms of my life as normal as possible, and keep as positive about the situation as I could. I wanted to remain as positive as I could, not only because that would help them stay positive and soften the blow of the news, but it would also help me keep my spirits up if everyone around me could remain positive.

When you help someone else, you end up helping yourself more.

This was key: If I was going to survive the thing mentally, and if my family and friends were going to survive it, then I had to learn how to stay on the positive mental path, independent of the physical path. I knew I was going to have to find a way to keep my routine as normal as possible and find a way to keep a stiff upper lip.

Keeping a normal routine was pretty easy: Three meals a day. Going out for a walk. Reading at night. Going out with friends. Keeping up my princess schedule of speaking engagements, dedications, my projects, and of course, my beauty routine. I even asked my doctor if I could continue getting injections of a botulinum toxin to soften some crow's feet around my eyes while on chemo! We are complicated creatures. There I was, doing everything I could to pump life into myself, yet I was asking if I could have injections of a neuro toxin to keep away a few squint lines. Princess priorities, I reckon. Fools R Us.

We'll Do What We Have to Do

As much as the daily routine was a no-brainer, the stiff upper lip was more challenging. Anyone here actually ever seen a stiff upper lip? I imagine it's what one's lip looks like when following my grandmother Lena Olian's advice, passed down to me from my father. When facing challenging times, Lena would always say, "We'll do what we have to do." That was good stuff from a woman with a stiff upper lip. It turned out that her advice, as well as her life, was a good role model for my future iteration as a breast cancer survivor.

My grandmother Lena was a beautiful woman until the day she passed at eighty-nine. She came to New York City from Grodno, Belorussia, with her family when she was around six. I grew up in Philadelphia, and my grandparents would come from New York to visit us. I could never figure out why Lena still had an accent, considering how young she had been when she came to the US. "Dahhlink. Dahhlink. You want a little nosh? Have a little nosh."

My father finally explained the accent. "She speaks Brooklynese."

Lena's "bad thing that happened" ended up being my big, helpful thing. It gave me courage and helped me through my mastectomy. If she were alive, she might very well have called that part finding the plus.

When Lena was a young mother, she was driving one of those big old cars, the kind in the 1930s with a huge steering wheel that looked like the captain's wheel on the Queen Mary. They had neither airbags nor seat belts back then. I never did find out exactly what happened, beyond the fact that when my father was about six, she was in a car accident. During that accident, the steering wheel crushed her chest completely, and she had to have her breasts removed. I don't know if there was any such thing as reconstruction back then, but if there was, she apparently didn't have it. I didn't know about the accident until she had passed away and I was way into adulthood. Lena never mentioned it, nor did any other family member. For her, it was just one of those we'll-do-what-we-have-to-do situations. She never seemed depressed or morose.

Because of my bout with breast cancer, I became interested in how Lena handled the accident and the loss of her breasts. My aunt (Lena's daughter) told me Lena had "just handled it." She told me Lena used to stuff her bra with cute little cotton things my aunt called "fuffies." Little did Lena know that her accident would one day help me handle my own difficult event.

On the day I was facing my mastectomy surgery, I carried my grandmother's legacy of doing what we have to do near to my heart. I kept thinking about her and how, just like royalty, she carried on without complaint. She had an aura of elegance that belied anything tragic in her life. And she certainly kept a stiff upper lip. Not only was that something possible of being passed on through the generations, it was being passed on to me when I needed it. I was grateful.

My goal in telling my kids was to find a way to reframe the news in a positive light.

Lena was so regal that her family called her The Queen. There was no snobbery to her behavior or demeanor, just an air of majesty. When she waited for the ambulance to come for what would be her last trip to the hospital, Lena polished her nails. And after she died, my mother put Lena's makeup kit in her coffin. It was Lena's equivalent of an ankh.

Lena was known as the peacemaker of the family, which is a very regal quality if you ask me. If there were any spats, Lena would be brought in to patch it up. She didn't start any squabbles either. One day she and PopPop were at some big hoo-haa fancy gala—a bar mitzvah, wedding, or fundraiser—and she must have been sitting at a peripheral table. Some *shmendrik* said, "Lena, are you upset that you are not at the head table?"

Lena replied without missing a beat, "Wherever I'm sitting, that *is* the head table."

Is that fabulous or is that fabulous? That queen knew the plus. She was sitting farther away from the loud obnoxious band!

As for telling the kids I was diagnosed with breast cancer, Howie and I talked it over, and he thought it was a good idea to use him as a buffer. He was going to break the news to the kids first. Or as Howie, a former college football player put it, he was going to run interference. That way, the kids could have whatever reaction they wanted to without worrying that they had to suck it up for my benefit. He also thought it would take the pressure off me. I could then talk to them after they digested the news.

I had my reservations about this approach because I was worried that if they couldn't see my face when he told them and they couldn't see that I was okay, it might be scarier for them. I wanted to tell and show them at the same time that I was fine. But I did also feel a sense of relief, and it took some pressure off me to have Howie break it to them.

When I probed Howie for information about what he was going to say to them, he wouldn't give me a clue. He merely said, "Don't worry about it. I said I'd handle it."

It ended up being a relief all right. Comic relief!

This is how it all went down. At 6:30 a.m., Howie was driving to Central Park on a race day. Howie does a lot of marathons and triathlons, and by a lot, I mean that as of this writing, he has finished eighteen marathons, over a hundred half-marathons, and twenty-four triathlons—including a full Ironman and three half-Ironmans—almost all of them within the last ten years. The kids are beginning to follow in his footsteps, pardon the pun. This day was one of the steps.

My youngest son, Max, was in the car with his girlfriend, Liz. He was twenty-six at the time. All three of them had done many races, and they had a routine—actually a tradition—for them. They always stopped for bagels on the way to the race. The kids stayed in the car while Howie hopped out to make the coffee and bagel run. Moveable feast. Meals on wheels.

But they broke from tradition that day. Why was this day different? Because on this day, Howie brought back not only bagels but something he never indulges in before a race—an assortment of glazed donut holes.

Howie hopped back in the car carrying the bag of bagels and donut holes, as well as coffee for each of them. "Hey! I've got bagels, and I also brought some donut holes!"

Yippee! Things were looking good. Howie took a donut hole for himself, passed the box back to the kids, and began driving again. The kids were eagerly and happily choosing their donut flavors, excited about the sweet detour from their healthier breakfast fare and never anticipating the bomb that was about to explode.

Howie took a bite of his donut hole and said, in a low voice, "By the way, your mother has breast cancer." Then, without skipping a beat, he exclaimed, "Wow! These chocolate glazed donut holes are delicious!"

That's how he broke the news to them. No lead-in. No buffer. No positivity. No pep talk. No nuthin'. According to Howie, Max and Liz were stunned.

That's running interference?

Max later told me that he was midair away from a bite of his donut hole when he got the news. And he had me in stitches as he reenacted the scene for me. He had scrunched up his face, thinking that he hadn't heard correctly. "Huh? What did Dad just say?" Max said that donut holes are ruined for him forever. (Which, by the way, is a big fat lie because I know that he recently brought a nice big box of them home for breakfast with Liz, who is now his wife. I'm super happy about that, and I hope you are too.)

When the race was over, Howie dropped off Max and Liz at their apartment in Jersey City and hightailed it over to my older son Harry and his fiancé (now wife) Amanda. I think he just straight up told them. According to Howie, they too were both stunned. Harry was too shocked to talk to me about it right away. He needed some time. For him, it was probably a good idea to have a buffer. But who knows? Maybe it would have been better for him to see my smiling face, making some jokes.

Perhaps there is no right or wrong way to tell the kids. Just tell them in a way that feels authentic to you, and then after a while, everybody acclimates.

The Power of Positive Words

When it came time for me to talk to the kids, I had my approach ready. I had decided I was going to choose positive, empowering words to describe the situation and what I was going to do about it. I knew the power of words and how one's choice of words can either empower or disempower.

I learned the power of words by accident early on in my legal career. I was given a very difficult assignment by my boss's boss's boss. I had no idea how to research, let alone handle, the assignment.

I was freaking out because I couldn't very well hand the assignment back to my boss's boss's boss and tell him I didn't know how to deal with it. I characterized the assignment to myself as a problem.

In case no one's noticed, something that is a problem . . . is problematic. Some thunderbolt of inspiration came to me and told me to look at the assignment as a challenge instead of as a problem. Almost immediately, I gained the clarity I needed to begin solving that challenge. That's when I realized that what we tell ourselves and how we tell it has an impact. By characterizing the issue as a challenge instead of a problem, we rise to it instead of feeling defeated.

The tactic of positive words that I had learned in my legal career was going to be deployed in my discussion with my kids. And I knew it would also help me keep a positive attitude for myself. I wanted to assure my kids that I was okay. As Howie wisely advised me at some point when I was frightened about breast cancer and wondering if I was okay, "You're okay if you say you're okay! Say you're okay!"

"I say I'm okay, and I'm okay," had become my mantra. The sheriff in town was going to kick cancer's butt!

When I talked to the kids, I used words that were empowering and positive. "I've got some good news and some challenging news. The good news is that the prognosis is excellent. The challenging news is that I have been diagnosed with breast cancer." Then I pronounced the law. "I'm going to kick cancer's butt!" That positive, strong statement felt invigorating. I felt a confidence coming from my own font of strength, and I knew it helped the kids tremendously.

In addition, I found even more positive angles to having breast cancer, and I talked about that with the kids. For example, this was going to give me a pant load of street cred for my happiness coaching practice.

If my prognosis had not been good, I would have said, "I've got some good news and some challenging news. The good news is that I'm facing a challenge the doctors are very familiar with, and I'm

The bottom line is you can't make doo-doo smell like roses, but you can buy some room spray.

under the best care possible. The challenging news is that I've been diagnosed with breast cancer."

As I said earlier, I believe there is no right or wrong way to break the news. Most likely, some ways work for some kids better than others. You can only do your best. In the end, what probably is best is what feels most authentic to you. It can sometimes help if you realize and articulate that lots of people have it a lot worse. My dad used to tell the parable about the man who complained about not having any shoes until he saw a man without any feet. It's up to you to figure out who those people are.

It will help you enormously if you endeavor to turn the challenge of breast cancer into a teaching moment. Ascribing meaning into this life event was a big positivity facilitator for me, and I decided to see it as a teaching moment for handling adversity. It was a gift I could give my kids to put in their pockets and take out as needed. I felt I had been given the opportunity to teach by example how to handle a difficult challenge and show my kids that trauma can be managed. None of us escapes life without hurdles. I was excited to turn what looked to me like a difficulty into a Life University lesson on how to weather storms. Course title: Handling the Crap Life Dishes Out 101.

My goal in the conversation was to make my diagnosis of breast cancer something other than the end of the world. To the extent I did that for my kids, I helped myself. I was teaching them that my getting through breast cancer was going to be about perspective and attitude, and this was how we were going to get though it together. When your family and friends see you having courage, they will have more courage.

Handling the News

A guy named Benjamin shared a story with me about what happened when his mom told him she had been diagnosed with breast cancer. Ben was a little kid when his mother was diagnosed with breast cancer. Ben told me he reacted to the news by asking, "What does that mean for me, Mom? Am I going to get cancer? And what will I do if you die?" Ben told me that to this day, as an adult, he feels guilty about his reaction. He was worried about what it meant for him and did not convey a sense of worry for his mom.

This is a wonderful window on what may be going on in our kids' minds when we break such news to them. When Benjamin told me his story and how guilty he felt about it, I was immediately able to console him because I knew how his mother would have felt. I explained how happy his mother must have been that he opened the dialogue to talk about it with her. I explained that one of the biggest fears we mothers have is that our children will be frightened and thrown into mental chaos. But the very fact that a child can ask questions and talk about it is very healthy. It creates an opportunity for the mother to discover what is actually going on in her kid's mind, which lets her know what issues hurt the most. Communication rules!

I have to admit, after I heard this story, I realized that another approach I could have taken with my kids was to ask them about their feelings and fears, as well as what questions they had. So you see, I was on a learning curve too. Perhaps my kids would not have wanted to talk about it, but I could have opened the door. But my kids had a fabulous sense of humor, and both of them recalibrated pretty quickly and went into humor mode with me. What I learned here was that other people don't always have as hard a time with something as you think they will.

And the way my kids handled the situation helped me immensely. My older son did something pretty funny—he shaved his beard in solidarity with me. That's right, not his head, his beard. "Go, Mom! I'm right there with ya." You'll understand how much funnier that "solidarity" is when you know that the "kid" gets five o'clock shadow at 10:00 a.m.

My kids adjusted pretty quickly to the news. I was more petrified about showing them my bald head then I was about telling them I had breast cancer. It's one thing to tell someone you've been diagnosed with breast cancer. In that moment, you might not look like anything is wrong, and it's not so scary for the other person. But the bald head seems so much a sign of trouble ahead in River City. Many of you might not experience this if you use the cold cap.

I didn't actually have to show them my bald head. I could have kept it under wraps. But I didn't want to make it a big deal and have to run and hide if they dropped by and I was going commando. When the big reveal came and I let the kids see my beautiful baldness, I was quite surprised and happy about everyone's reaction. Harry was neither shocked nor dismayed. He was excited to discover how much we looked alike. "Mom, you look like me! It's like looking at myself!" That was pretty funny.

Max, my younger son, adjusted pretty quickly after the donut debacle. And we both laughed pretty hard when we reminded each other how breast cancer was "so great" because I was going to have a lot more street cred with my "How to be Royally Happy" seminars. Street cred became our inside joke and a buzz phrase to thumb our noses at breast cancer, as if to say, "You can *try* to hurt me, but fat chance!"

My brother bolstered my confidence by citing all the models and hip gals walking around New York City sporting bald heads on purpose. He assured me that it could be a very chic, very cool look. My husband's reaction was amazing and soulful. He told me I looked beautiful. He also told me that I had a really nicely shaped head. What a lovely thing to say! He also bolstered my confidence with the reconstruction. "You look great, and now your back won't hurt when you get older." He took a page from Fanny's playbook, making everything a plus.

The moral of the story here is that how well *you* handle the situation may be determinative of how well others take the news. Also, breaking the news could very well go better than you fear. And you never know, you might end up laughing about it like we did. Everything is a plus. There is *always* a plus.

Here's a funny take on another plus factor of my breast cancer. Max went for a job interview. The recruiters asked him what his biggest challenge in life was. His answer? He said it was when he found out his mom had breast cancer. He said it was hard going to work every day in the beginning and that I was his hero because talking to me, you'd never know what I was going through. Max said, "You know, Mom, I think that might be one reason I got the job!" That gave both of us a good laugh. I told you, everything is a plus!

Different family members may handle the news differently. To the extent a princess can find something positive to say, even if it's "We are a family, and as a family, we will find resilience to face the challenges, whatever they are," that will bring some strength and some light to the situation.

Benjamin's mom handled telling him about her cancer brilliantly. "Whatever happens to me," she said, "even if I die, I will always be with you. I will always protect you. I will always be in your eyes, your mind, and your cells. I will always be looking down from the heavens and be with you." That helped him immensely.

I thought of Benjamin's mother when talking to a new friend of mine who had breast cancer when her kids were small. She told me that her fear of leaving them and the accompanying worry about their fear was the most frightening part of it. She didn't know how to handle that. Luckily, she had a good prognosis too, so she was "just" dealing with her fear and not the harsh prospect of probable demise from breast cancer. If probable early demise had been the case, I think Benjamin's mom's words would have been very comforting to her little children.

The bottom line is you can't make doo-doo smell like roses, but you can buy some room spray. If you decide you need to deal with the issue and you have young kids, in my opinion, the more you can convey the positive points in the situation facing you, the hopeful points, the better they will feel. There is always something to dwell on to give us hope.

For instance, when I first found out that my cancer was not confined to the breast but had already gotten into my lymph nodes, I became very afraid of dying. As I said earlier, I tried to think of all the things that were hopeful in my situation. It brought me hope to think that I had doctors who really cared about me and who knew what they are doing. I found it hopeful to think that modern medicine is very powerful. I found it hopeful to dwell on the fact that scientists and researchers were finding new ways to make people better all the time. I also found hope in the fact that miracles happen every day. I sought out stories of people who had been very sick and then miraculously got well. It can happen. It was not beyond possibility. Those thoughts were very helpful to me. I found it very hopeful to focus on the fact that I was alive *that* day, and that nobody had a window on their future next day. I had as much as anybody else.

I have read ideas from women who have not had a good prognosis about how they have handled the situation with their young children. Some of them write letters to their children to be given on different occasions. Some of them create videos telling of their love and offering encouragement so the kids will have something from them through-out their lifetime. I know this sounds very grim, but I would have chosen to do that in their situation, so I am passing that on to you. It would have encouraged me to know that I was leaving something for my kids that they would always have and which might help them.

I would try to include something uplifting, even humorous, so that the children would have a happy memory mixed in with the sadness. That would be a true teaching moment.

It recently dawned on me that the word *encourage* has the French word *coeur*—heart—in it. Heart. I thought it might be helpful to come up with some ways to encourage the kiddies, by fortifying them and strengthening them. My particular method to fortify and encourage them with heart was to shelter them with an umbrella of positivity and humor. Through Benjamin, I learned that another way to fortify them could be by asking them how they felt and addressing their concerns.

For me, the object in breaking the news to my kids was to find a positive angle, and I had a plan that felt comfortable to me. But you don't have to figure out how to handle breaking the news to your children by yourself. Sometimes it's helpful to seek professional help. At least, it's something to consider. Hospitals often have social workers, chaplains, and other resources, and they may also be able to refer you to professionals skilled in providing professional guidance. Don't be afraid to get help.

A princess always considers the well-being of her kingdom, and that's what you're doing here, royal friend.

Meaning-Mindedness

I have already mentioned above that using the breast cancer diagnosis and treatment journey as a teaching moment for kids can inherently help you by giving meaning to the experience. I'd like to dive into that issue of meaning a little deeper because it's a biggie when it comes to happiness.

I first heard of Viktor Frankl's iconic book, *Man's Search for Meaning*, from Fanny. Frankl was a Jewish German psychiatrist who survived the atrocities of the Auschwitz concentration camp during WWII. His parents, a brother, and his young wife perished.

Fanny told me she read Viktor Frankl's book over and over again. It helped her deal with the trauma she had lived through.

Frankl tried to minister to fellow prisoners in the death camp. Again and again, he talked about trying to invigorate inner fortitude, and the first thing he believed was needed for that was a goal for living, which he saw as being critical for survival.[8] Because their future was so bleak and their chances for survival so small, Frankl realized that he needed to help them—and himself—find a new way of looking at life. They needed to find meaning, but it had to come from a different focus. He realized that people in despair might be helped if they found meaning in the way they faced up to the suffering.[9]

The idea of creating a *why* to live based on the *how* of handling your suffering recently showed up for me in real time and on real terms. A cherished friend of mine told me doctors had given her two years to live—five years ago. Medical discoveries had been helping her beat the odds, but living life in her usual vibrant and full way had become a profound challenge. And how long her "reprieve" would last was unknown.

At the same time, her daughter was facing her own dangerous, life-threatening battle. And as every parent knows, when your child is facing anything that could take their life, the concern about that is even more profound than concern about your own life. My friend has to continually fight to keep her health, both physical and mental. She told me that all she wants to do is to age with grace and face her future with grit, compassion, and grace.

It dawned on me that perhaps that is exactly what Frankl was talking about. The suffering in my friend's situation is profound and protracted. Yet she has found a way to keep going instead of giving up, possibly because she found an aim within her suffering.

As I mentioned earlier, I too found an aim to my suffering. I looked forward to being able to show my kids that even when life is a crap sandwich, you can find a way to go on. I put this concept in the forefront of my mind and focused on it a lot when I found myself spiraling down. It helped me rise up and remember that if I could help my kids, or my friends, or someone else get through the suffering by showing them they could still find joy, then it was worth at least some of the admission cost.

Miracle-Mindedness

There is a powerful life force that attaches in an attitude shift when one finds the "why" to live. Losing all hope for one's future can have devastating consequences. We have to find something to give us hope, some reason to find meaning for going on, even under dire circumstances, or we risk losing our will to live. Suddenly losing our will to live can result in an immune system that stops supporting us. Hope can come from knowing that new methods of diagnosis and treatment are developed every day. These could be considered miracles. They just happen to be miracles we can see.

Lest you think that miracle-mindedness is for woo-woo people and wusses, think again. Brainiac and rational thinker Albert Einstein believed you could either look at everything as a miracle or nothing as one. And the Sufi poet Rumi said that we should never lose hope because there are miracles. I don't believe this means that you can sit back and do nothing to help yourself because you are going to let a miracle do all the heavy lifting. No, you keep doing what you need to do while remaining receptive to a miracle. Trust in your Higher Power but water your houseplants.

Being receptive to miracles is just another bullet in your ammunition belt to help you remain hopeful in the face of dire news. I find it is helpful to keep my mind open to what other religions have to say on topics I am interested in. What resonates, I take. What doesn't resonate, I leave.

I am convinced that miracles happen because every time I think of the birth of a child, or the fig trees and delphinium in my garden, or Lalo, my French bulldog, I know that their very existence is a miracle. So what's the big deal about one more?

Meaty, Mighty Might-Mindedness

Another tool for reframing things is the concept of the meaty, mighty might. That is about breaking through the bleak unknown when the future is scary. For sure, things *might* look bad, but on the other hand, things *might* be okay. There is a lot of meaty might packed into that thought. Here's how I stumbled on this idea.

The mother of a colleague was seriously ill and frightened. My colleague was trying to calm her mother's fears. When her mother would get in frantic mode and start ticking off all the reasons why she felt the situation looked bleak and why she felt there was very little hope, my colleague would exclaim, "But things *might* be okay." In other words, *there is some space for a good outcome.* So even if the doctors are saying this one thing, this other thing *might* be true. Even if the doctors say things look bad, things *might* turn out okay. This is true. Nobody knows the future for sure.

Just this little ray of real, true, and authentic *possibility* of hope for a positive outcome turned everything around for the fear factor for her mom. And so far, she is okay. So far, the meaty, mighty might is right!

The power inherent in positive possibilities should not be discounted. It is really important when it comes to a serious illness. We must live in these possibilities to keep hope in front of our noses. Of course, we should not neglect the actions we need to take to keep ourselves healthy and go forward for a positive outcome. Again, as with miracle-mindedness, we wouldn't say, "Okay, I *might* be okay, so I don't have to take my medication." The point is to retain your reason and horse sense while not discounting the power of meaty, mighty might thinking.

We must go forward and stoke the bits of hope that are available to us rather than pour cold water on the embers of positivity with our outlook on life. The evidence is clear that looking for the positive and finding optimism even in bleak circumstances is not a fool's journey. Or as I like to say, optimism is optimizing your chances for a better outcome.

Optimism creates psychological resilience while you are pursuing the better outcome. Indeed, I have found that if I am optimistic, I pursue courses that actually make what I want to happen, happen.

For example, there are many times I have given it all I've got while running to catch a train that, by all train schedule timetables, I am *surely* not going to make. I am just pure and simply too late. I cannot count how many times I would have missed the train if I had given up. But because I *didn't* give up, because I tried anyway in spite of what it looked like on the clock, I made the train. For sure, a long shot. And I wasn't going to be thirty minutes late. I'm talking a few minutes late. But I certainly would not have made the train if I had given up when things looked bleak.

I recently heard about a woman with stage four ovarian cancer whose doctor had given up hope on a cure. He had told her to get her affairs in order. She was cured by a novel form of treatment at another hospital. That's the meaty, mighty might doing the happy dance.

Choosing Not to Break It to Your Kids

I have read stories about women who actually never told their kids. The kids were quite young and the women did not want to frighten them. They wore wigs after chemo and went to work as usual, and their kids never knew. So if that is something you want to do, there is precedent for that. I can't advise you on that because you know your kids, and I don't.

I believe kids are a lot more resilient than we think, and after the initial shock, if you seem okay and remain positive, I believe there is a good chance they will be okay too. It's a really good incentive for you to try to remain positive.

But there is something more to consider. A friend taught me that if there is a big family secret you keep from your children, they will pick up on the fact that something is going on anyway. And because you don't tell them what the secret is, the secret itself gives them fear. In other words, if there is something happening that is so bad you can't tell them, they might be even more scared because you can't tell them. That's just something to consider.

Breaking the News to Other Family Members

Howie was in on the jig from the get-go. The doctors basically broke it to the two of us together. It was extremely helpful to have him with me in the earliest stages of investigation. I was lucky that Howie was able to absorb the shock pretty quickly. He told me his attitude was to do whatever he could to be supportive and make me feel as comfortable and confident as possible. He was focused on my well-being and wanted me to make choices that would be best for my health.

Of course, I was worried that if I had a mastectomy, my physical attractiveness and desirability might diminish in his eyes. Here's where you have to remember that our imaginings are often much worse than reality. Howie's reaction before and after the surgery was and continues to be incredibly encouraging to me. Howie told me he felt bad for *me*, but he didn't feel bad for *himself*. Would he prefer that I had my old boobs, the ones that had nipples attached to them? Yeah. I would have liked them back too, along with their nerve endings. But Howie's attitude was, if that's what it is, that's what it is. I was the one that was going through it. It wasn't his place to be upset or annoyed by it. It was his place to accept it. He told me he never felt he was losing out on anything. And it turns out that he totally likes the way I look now.

The moral of the story is, don't necessarily expect some big drama from your partner around mastectomy surgery. In any event, give both you and any partner time to let the blow of the news settle. I know in my own mind, time helped normalize the shock of it all.

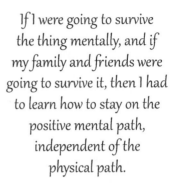

If I were going to survive the thing mentally, and if my family and friends were going to survive it, then I had to learn how to stay on the positive mental path, independent of the physical path.

As for my sister, I informed her immediately. Even if she weren't a doctor, I would have told her for her emotional support and her brainpower. Additionally, I enlisted the support of my brother from the beginning, and he was a huge source of emotional support. They both came to many doctor appointments with me to help me decipher the mumbo jumbo, and they listened to my fears in between.

What I learned is that smarty pants or no smarty pants, it is super hard to make decisions about these medical matters by yourself. And that's another really good reason to break it to the grown-up-ish members of your family. To the extent that you can bring a family member (or friend) to some of the initial appointments, it is a good idea to do that. They can not only provide emotional support, they will be a second set of ears. Half the time, I couldn't retain or process what the doctors said because I was so frightened. Perhaps even more disconcerting, it was super easy for me to retain the bad information and practically not even hear (or process) the good stuff. You are going to need all pistons firing to make the important decisions. Bringing someone along with you is one way to help you retain and analyze the necessary information. I really felt I needed my sister for her medical help, brainpower, and support. I wanted Howie and my brother for their brainpower and emotional support as well.

And then there was the issue of my elderly parents. What about them? My mom had dementia, so we didn't tell her. But did I really have to tell my ninety-three-year-old dad? I was in a conundrum over that decision. We had a sibling powwow. My sister and brother thought we should, and I ended up agreeing. But here are the thoughts that were going on in my now iconically fried brain.

My dad was 100 percent still with it. I knew he and Mom had friends and family who had died of breast cancer. Dad was going to know all the dangers, but he might not know about all the medical progress. In particular, one of my parents' best friends had died of breast cancer many years earlier.

I enlisted the opinions of my sister, my brother, and Howie about whether to tell Dad. We all debated it. I figured he was going to know something was up when I had to wear a wig. My brother and sister thought we should tell him because if he found out some other way, he might be hurt.

We chose the running interference approach. My brother would break it to him on our next collective visit. When my sister, my brother, and I went to visit Dad and Mom, my sister and I wandered off by ourselves while my brother stayed in Dad's room to talk. After my brother told him, it broke my heart to see him sitting in his wheelchair with a worried face. He looked teary-eyed. But I helped by making jokes with him, and he quickly saw that I was doing okay and not falling apart, which dissipated the cloud.

Here's a little perspective. Over a very short period of time, even bad news tends to normalize. This happened with my dad. You might find yourself and others joking about the situation. No big surprise on that one with my family! Right before I was going to have my bilateral mastectomy, Dad made a joke that the surgery wasn't really that big a deal. He said the surgery was really like taking off two big moles! I thought that this perspective was fantastic and hysterical. The joking helped him, and it helped me too. And you know what?

In a way, he was right. The two lumps of breast tissue are like two big moles!

I should have expected this reaction. My dad was the most positive person I ever knew. As a kid, he was our alarm clock for getting up in the morning to go to school. He would have a big smile on his face, emanating positive energy as he clapped his hands together at the three kids sleeping in their three respective rooms and declared, "Rise and shine!" and "Up and at 'em!" Sometimes he'd be whistling. I'd say that was a good start to the day for most of my young life.

I was diagnosed in January, and Dad passed in October. I was totally surprised that I found a sense of comfort that Dad knew about my breast cancer and knew that I was doing well. I feel his presence on a daily basis. It's a matter of energy. That is what I feel, an unbreakable bond of connection. It feels like he is resonant and reachable in the ethers. I don't have to send him a message about what is going on in my health because I am assured that he knew while he was earthbound. I am eternally grateful that I had been able to talk and joke with him about it. He made peace with it. I saw that with my eyes and my heart.

The question of whether to tell my precious, beautiful mom was easy. At the time, Mom had a pretty bad case of dementia, so there was no use telling and worrying her. Although she is in full-blown dementia now, at the beginning stages of my breast cancer diagnosis, we could still talk to her, and she would get the drift of a conversation, even if she couldn't really negotiate the daily doings of life. My concern was that she would understand in the moment what was going on, which would give her unnecessary pain, but she wouldn't remember by the end of the day, or even moments later. And she couldn't help me anyway, so there was no point in telling her.

If my mom did not have dementia, it would have been extremely hard to tell her because she'd spent a lifetime as an inveterate worrier. Mom had a kind of perverse idea that if she worried about something, the thing she worried about wouldn't happen. I could just imagine how much mental real estate would have been taken up in her mind if I had to tell her about my breast cancer diagnosis, the surgery, the chemo, and everything else.

But I would have liked to have been able to tell my beautiful, brilliant, kind-hearted yet strong mother. My mom and I were always very close. She always had good advice for me, and I always felt safe with her. From the very earliest memories I have of school, where achieving good grades was super important to me, when I told my mother my fears that I wouldn't do well on any particular test, she would always say, "Don't worry. Just do the best that you can." That always calmed me down. I felt that with the cancer thang, she would have found a way to calm me down just because she would have wanted to help me. But even if she didn't show me her worry, I know she would have done her worrying in private.

Mom loved me so much, no matter what. Those were some of the last words she told me before she fell into really bad dementia, during which she didn't speak much on a proactive basis. We said we loved one another no matter what. And we both knew that was true. I would have liked to have Mom in my corner, but on some level, I think she has been. A mom is a mom, no matter what.

Look Ahead to the Future

When my parents were transferring from their independent living center to the medical center, we three adult kids took it upon ourselves to clean out their apartment. They both skipped the assisted living phase that was available there. That's the "Do not pass go. Do not collect $200" of the senior living set. There were a couple of huge bookshelves with lots of books on them. Their furniture, most of which was antiques, was auctioned off. As for the books, it was hard to choose what to save and what to leave for the movers.

I don't know why we didn't ask for guidance about which books Dad wanted to save, which is something I regret. There was such limited space where he was going, and we were aggressive about getting rid of stuff. I recognized the prayer books from synagogue. One was Dad's and one was Mom's. I saved them both. My brother set aside his medical books. But I found out later that one important book escaped us: Dad's father's Hebrew prayer book. Either we saw it and didn't recognize it for what it was or we didn't see it.

The movers came and went. Later, my unassuming dad, who never asked us for anything and never asked us to do anything for him, asked about one thing only. He wanted to know where his father's prayer book was. Oh my gosh! My heart sank, and I felt horrible! The one darn book that Dad asked about, the one and only thing he asked for, the only book that might have been a source of comfort to him in his last years . . . we had not saved.

We all searched among the books that were left piled on the floor of his old room, but this golden family treasure wasn't among them. When I told my dad, he said without the slightest bit of gloom, anger, or agitation, "Oh well, we have to look forward and not look back."

He said it just like that—just as a matter of fact. His priority was making sure we felt okay.

Thus, he pulled out of his bag of tricks a life lesson. He pulled out Lena's "We'll do what we have to do." He had to look forward and not look back, not lament the loss of this family prayer book. It was just one loss among many: the loss of his life the way it had been; the loss of good food because his sense of taste diminished; the loss of things unknown to anyone but him.

That is a wonderful way to look at life and the events that happen. Just look forward. Don't look back. This was how my father handled just about everything when he had to leave his old life behind, and it became a lesson for me about how I should handle my situation and how to share the information about it with others. And leave it to my dad, his perspective was biblical.

The Bible has a brilliant story in it about what happens when you look back. It's the story of Lot's wife, whom some call Edith. Edith was told not to look back at the city of Sodom. When she did, she turned into a pillar of salt. I take this story to mean that if a person looks back, he or she might become like a pillar of salt by crying copious tears. We must do what it takes to survive mentally, as well as physically. Practicality rules. I learned it from the best.

You can keep this future-oriented perspective in mind when breaking it to other family members. It can help everyone if you keep a perspective that you are looking toward the future and not wallowing in the past. There were times when I had a palace pop-up pity party and longed for the me I used to be. But then I quickly recalibrated because, as I've opined before, what am I gonna do with that? I used positive psychology techniques to reframe the situation. Why long for what was when I could focus on the "new and improved" me? If there was a "yeah, but," I reminded myself that I got to live.

Look to the future!

Friends and Strangers

Contrary to what you might think, not everybody gets all choked up when they hear that someone they know has a cancer diagnosis. Some people can muster humor right away. When I told a dentist friend of mine that I was worried about whether the shot I got from my oncologist every six months to help address bone density loss due to my treatment would affect my jaw, a possible side effect, he joked, "You've got bigger things to worry about."

I'm being a tad tongue-in-cheek here, but humor me. Here's a dirty little wink-wink secret that no one talks about: When people find out you're being treated for breast cancer, they start treating you like you're a celebrity. People smile at you more. People seem to start liking you more. In stores, clerks sometimes give you discounts. When I dropped the C-bomb in one store, the sales person started rummaging through papers to find coupons and discounts that only applied if you used a credit card, which I wasn't using. What a perk! People want to buy you things. I got all sorts of cancer booty: necklaces, books, fun baskets, coloring books, and beautiful boxes of multi-colored pencils. People didn't know what to throw at me, but I appreciated it all.

Sometimes your treatments will be a great excuse to weasel out of chores. If your kids, husband, or any other person asks you to do something you don't feel like doing—walking the Tibetan mastiff, cleaning the bathroom "throne," making (reservations for) dinner, or anything else—use this trick. Bat your eyelashes (if you still have them) and say in your sweetest, most vulnerable baby voice, "I caaaaan't. I've got caaaaan-cer." This works like a charm!

How Friends Can Help

Friends can be a great source of help during these trying times. At first, I didn't want to tell my friends because I was concerned that they might run away from me out of fear. Howie's grandfather, who came from the Ukraine, used to say that everybody is your friend until you're sick. Maybe it was just some Old World thing, but it stuck in the back of my mind and came out to strike fear in my heart. I think that some people are genuinely afraid to go through the pain of losing you, so they distance themselves. Perhaps there is a stigma against people who have an illness, especially a serious one. I also believe that some people are afraid because the illness cuts too close to home, and they are afraid for themselves.

If some people do distance themselves from you, I want you to do your best to forgive them. The last thing you need is another burdensome emotion to drag around. Don't be too quick to judge them or to jump to the conclusion that because they flaked out on you, they are not your true friends. Maybe they are not, but maybe they are. Do yourself a major favor: Don't abandon them in return, don't write them off, and don't become bitter. Bitterness won't help in your own healing journey. Bitterness prevents you from flying light emotionally and from feeling good inside. And above all, do not seek revenge. There's an old saying that if you want to seek revenge, dig two graves. It's not that they don't care. Most likely they can't handle it.

I know this seems counterintuitive, but it's true. People are funny birds. They don't always act how we expect them to or how we would react. Give them the benefit of the doubt.

The moral of the story is that we are all mere mortals with our faults, frights, and foibles. You never know what people go through. Your illness might resonate with them in a way that they cannot handle. Perhaps they lost a loved one when they were very young, and they absolutely cannot deal with this issue in a mature way. Give them some slack.

Here's a strategy for giving people the benefit of the doubt and preventing you from hardening your heart to the world: Tell yourself that they are doing the best they can. Most of the time, we are all just doing the best we can with what we have and where we are. A boss of mine used to say, "You go with what you've got on a given day." That's what people do.

In the meantime, many of your friends will be totally in your face wanting to help. This is a wonderful thing. I was lucky. Most of my friends reacted in a most supportive way. Many wanted to visit me. Some took me to lunch. Many wanted to bring me some little gift or distraction in the face of my impending chemotherapy. These were a source of comfort as well as beautiful to look at and play with. When I look at my stash of gifts, they represent the beautiful souls who brought them.

Here's an APB to your friends: Don't run away from your breast cancer sisters (and brothers). You are not a bad person if you do, so forgive yourselves in advance. But try your best to connect, even if it's just a phone call to see how they are doing. Reaching out so they realize they are not alone in this world is a big deal. And if they are afraid of being shunned, your call will reassure them that you are still there for them, that you haven't skipped town on the next stagecoach. You are part angel, you know. This is one of the easier assignments to get those wings of yours while you are still an earthling!

Here are some ideas for helping friends who have been diagnosed with breast cancer. Offer to:

- go wig or scarf shopping with her,
- accompany her on a chemo session or doctor's appointment,
- take her out to lunch,
- plan a day at a museum,
- go with her to a comedy show,
- get tickets to the theater,
- go to an indoor or outdoor concert with her,
- take her on a fancy croissant and chocolates coffee break,
- take her for ice cream (and insist on rainbow sprinkles),
- host a mimosa brunch,
- help with the kids,
- host a coloring book party,
- go on a walk in the park with her,
- take her on a trip down the shore if it's nearby,
- go kayaking together,
- take a walk along a canal or pond with her,
- host a positivity book club,
- browse a vintage bookstore with her,
- go with her to a beauty store (like Sephora or Ulta) and get makeup demos,

- play cards or board games (with or without wine) with her and other friends,
- plan a day at the races,
- go to a garden show with her,
- get mani-pedis together,
- watch a funny movie by yourselves or with others,
- do yoga together in home or at a class,
- host a pajama party sleepover.

If you want to buy little gifts for her, cute little necklaces that are meaningful or little bracelets with charms are fun. Coloring books with mandalas or flower and nature scenes are nice as an activity to take one's mind off of chemo. A book that you think she will like is great too.

Help Yourself by Helping Your Friends and Family

Here's another key, and this is a critical piece of the self-help strategy: We are comforted and helped when we comfort and help others. The biggest gift you can give yourself is giving *of* yourself to those who want to help you. Allow them to meet with you. Allow them to give you what they need to give you. But also allow them to *not* give to you if that's what they need. Allow them the grace of space if they can't handle the situation. If they are a friend, help yourself by helping them still be your friend. If they are a family member, help yourself by continuing to love them.

In fact, a little love and understanding all around—for yourself, for your family, and for your friends—is not only a way to stay positive through your cancer journey, it is a major princess tool for staying positive throughout the entire life journey. It's the royal secret sauce to the pudding of life, and now you have the recipe too.

10

Becoming Permission-Minded

A princess can defy the gravity of gravity by
giving herself permission to be happy.
–Princess Diane von Brainisfried

There's a trick to living well: Give yourself permission to live well! So much of what we experience in life is related to our internal self-talk. When I was first diagnosed with breast cancer, I had a whole paradigm built around what that meant. It included being and looking sick. It included not having fun anymore. My mind was like Scrooge visiting the ghosts of Christmas past, present, and future, only never having that marvelous Christmas morning epiphany. It was never waking up from the nightmare and never having that second chance. But I did wake up—because I decided to wake up.

Confucius said, "We have two lives, and the second begins when we realize we only have one." What happened to Scrooge when he woke up? He got a second chance at life. How? He gave himself a second chance. He gave himself permission to change and live from the best version of himself. When Scrooge was visited by the three ghosts, he got a shocker. He saw what he had made of his life, and he didn't like it one bit. The morning after the visitation, he threw open the windows and made a decision to be someone different: someone he liked; someone other people liked; someone generous of spirit; someone with joy in his heart who was joyfully dedicated to spreading joy.

First, though, Scrooge had to change the way he looked at himself. He had to believe that he was the type of person who could be joyous and spread joy. Otherwise, he would have gone back to his same old Scroogely habits, which included being a stingy, mean, bitter curmudgeon. He had to change his identity. To do so, he had to change his *mind* about himself, change his *habits* of thought. He had to change his paradigm of what Scroogeness meant.

Similarly, I had to change my mind about my identity as a breast cancer patient to avoid adopting the habits that matched my paradigm of being a breast cancer patient. And instead of the word *patient*, I could have substituted the word *victim*, because that's how I felt. But I didn't want to be or see myself as a victim. So instead of being blue or depressed, I worked on habits that helped me stay happy and live joyously. I was determined not to become the paradigm of breast cancerness. But the first thing I had to do was live in a permission-minded way. I had to give myself permission to be happy and joyous. I had to give myself permission to normalize my world. I had to name it and claim it.

But there's often something sneaky that happens when we make decisions: a big "but." And that big but is how?

The Big But: How?

The first time I realized the existence and importance of the big-but-how issue was as a new voice student, years ago, with a voice teacher I'll call Mr. Bark. Mr. Bark often told me that to reach the high notes, I needed to get my epiglottis down. There were three problems with that request: I didn't know *what* my epiglottis was. I didn't know *where* my epiglottis was. And when I did learn what and where my epiglottis was, I didn't know *how* to put my epiglottis down. How was I supposed to do that?

There's a trick to living well: Give yourself permission to live well!

You can't just tell someone to put their epiglottis down but not tell them how to do it. That would be like telling a novice cook who wants to make a soufflé that she needs to separate ten eggs but not telling her how to separate the eggs. Separate them how? Put five whole eggs in one bowl and five eggs in another? Of course not. There's a technique for separating eggs. You make a slight crack in the egg by hitting it against a sharp, thin surface so the eggshell is horizontally cracked but not yet spilling. Then you carefully pull apart the shells, letting the clear goo drop into one bowl and the yellow yolk goop drop into another bowl. Voila! Eggs separated.

Luckily, I didn't stay with that voice teacher very long. The next superstars I studied with never mentioned the word *epiglottis*. Instead, they gave me all kinds of tips to keep my throat open in the back so the sound had the greatest amount of freedom, openness, and resonance. And of course, just telling me to keep my throat open in the back was a way better *how* than telling me to get my epiglottis down.

"Make believe the roof of your mouth is the steeple of a church," my new voice teachers would say, or "Think of an inner yawn," or "Keep a little smile inside," or "Pretend you are sipping inward through a straw." All of these suggestions helped me acquire the technique of singing freely in the upper ranges. I was probably getting my epiglottis down. Didn't know. Didn't care. And that's the name of *that* tune. Tra-la-la.

I made the decision to give myself permission to be happy and joyous instead of being a victim after my diagnosis of breast cancer. But I still needed to know how to do that. How could I actualize that permission? How could I create the habit of happiness under these circumstances?

I had many strategies for being happy when I wasn't walking around with breast cancer in the picture. I was already writing and giving workshops about that. But would I be able to apply what I knew to my new situation? I didn't have anyone to show me the way. I didn't have a new paradigm for happiness with breast cancer to deflect me from the scary paradigm in my head. I had some learning to do.

It turns out that many of the techniques for creating happiness in life don't change with changing situations. I just had to *apply* them in the new situations. Along the way, necessity did teach me some additional happiness strategies, bless necessity's little heart.

All of us have accumulated wisdom for handling life's crises. You may not recognize it, but you *do* have this wisdom. Maybe you ate one too many caviar-filled blinis and couldn't fit into your ball gown. Maybe the royal goldfish died. Maybe your older princess sister picked on you for licking your fingers and smacking your chops when the basket of fried chicken was finger lick'n good. You learned tricks and strategies on your own to deal with life's knotty problems. You knew a good seamstress and you let the dress out. You bought a new goldfish and named it Bob's Your Uncle. You dropped your sister off at the palace gate and *then* chowed down on the takeout. Your own resourcefulness can be called upon by looking back at how you solved problems in the past. You have it in you naturally. You did it then, and you can do it now. Don't forget that you own your own princess power!

Being diagnosed with cancer is a pretty big shocker. Even a princess can get knocked off her gilded perch with this one. It's emotionally upsetting, to say the least. After giving myself permission to be happy, I wracked my brain to pull up strategies of positivity and optimism I already knew.

It can be a real struggle in life to constantly fight against "what is." But it's also easier said than done to stop that fighting. Sometimes having a handy expression of worldly wisdom in your silk-embroidered pocket can help. One of those expressions is this: It is what it is. Usually you have to stick a sigh at the beginning. "Ahh . . . it is what it is." I practiced that sigh, and usually muttered what followed it. There's a saying I really like that I picked up along my travels somewhere: We must learn to accept the is-ness of things. It is what it is.

Just as it's a mistake to think that you can't fight city hall, it's a mistake to think you can't fight other challenges in life. When it comes to city hall, sometimes you can fight it and sometimes you can't. The same goes for other challenges. It's important to understand this when the fight drains your energy and leaves you more stressed than necessary. How was I going to fight the fact that I was diagnosed with breast cancer? That was a fact. I just had to accept the is-ness of this newest iteration of my life.

Learn to accept the is-ness of things and the difficulties of life that you cannot control will be a lot easier to take. Keep your eye on the prize: peace in your soul, not a piece of your soul.

There's another expression that helps one grapple with this new upside-down life: the new normal. At a time when things seem anything but normal, it's a nice grounding expression because it has the word *normal* in it. It's normalizing. Things aren't so upside down if there's the word normal in it. And everyone likes something new. Put those two words together and we've got some of our happiness mojo back. New + Normal = New Normal.

Knowing that the collective consciousness of wisdom already had my back was comforting. Being the positive princess I am, after I caught my breath from my diagnosis, I wanted to venture out one step further with my sick inner child tucked under my arm and into the "it is what it is" and the "is-ness" of my new normal. I wanted my "is" to be happy, positive, and optimistic. But how? That mother with the sick child under her arm, how is she able to be happy? Is it even possible? It didn't seem so. Resolute? Maybe. Functional? I'll give her that on a good day. And those are two really positive qualities. I would never knock functional and resolute. It can be a big deal sometimes just to put one foot in front of the other and breathe.

But I was worried. I didn't want to go through this experience—and possibly life—merely functional and resolute. I was going to have to find new mental tactical maneuvers to live a happy, positive, optimistic life. It felt like I was going to have to find a way to up my game.

Here's why. The diagnosis of breast cancer made me feel freakish, as if an alien had taken up residence inside me. As if I didn't know myself. As if there was some little green monster inside of me turning on cellular activity that I had no knowledge of and making me something that I was not or someone I had never conceived myself to be.

And there's another thing that loomed over me: my own pre-fabricated paradigm of what a cancer patient should be like. The crap we can come up with in our own heads is crazy. I didn't think I was "allowed" to be happy. It felt like I was disrespecting the gravity of the situation—defying the gravity of the gravity. It seemed to me that someone in my situation did not really have permission to be laughing, playful, and carefree. How could I be carefree with this *sick* kid under my arm?

It's kind of like when you're reading *Bambi*. You know that Bambi's mom bites the dust. You don't really feel like you have permission from the universe to instigate a tickle fight during little junior's bedtime story time when you know what's coming. Same thing when you're reading about Peter Rabbit, whom you know will soon be facing down the barrel of Mr. McGregor's shotgun. We know the storyline.

I felt kind of like that. Even though I didn't feel sick, I knew something not so pretty was coming. I wondered how I was allowed to call myself happy when I was a member of the Big C club. How was I allowed to say I was happy when there was a stranger inside me doing mean things to my innards? In a sense, I didn't feel whole. I felt fragmented, split asunder into two parts, mind and body. And the body was doing its own thing.

Then I said to myself, the heck with that! Time for a new way of thinking! Out with the old paradigm, in with the new! If I were going to be able to maintain a happiness homeostasis, I was going to have to give myself *permission* to have a tickle fight reading *Bambi* or smile at Peter Rabbit in the garden. Bang! That's all, folks!

Here's the key: It's our life, and we get to rewrite the script. The new script is called *The Great in Spite of and the Big I Don't Care Who Says So*. If I gave myself permission, I could be happy in spite of whatever was coming my way. Who said I couldn't? I don't care! This was transformational.

I remembered what my yoga teacher had said: It's not what's happening to you that's important, it's what you tell yourself is happening to you that's important. I was going to have to get into the habit of talking to myself differently. I needed to write a new inner script. What I was telling myself about what was going on was going to have to be different.

It wasn't about going into denial or going all-out ostrich and sticking my head in the sand. I didn't even think ostriches really did that. But more importantly, there were ways of talking about a situation, characterizing a situation, in a more positive way. The new script would reframe how I looked at myself and talked to myself about what was happening to me. For example, the hunter who shot Bambi's mom had a case of Montezuma's revenge and never made it out hunting that day. Mr. McGregor had terrible aim and couldn't shoot an elephant from ten feet away. Peter Rabbit had a bulletproof vest, pepper spray, and his own private getaway drone. Rewrites, princess! Rewrites!

Permission to Accept Personal Sherpas

There's a time in life when we have to make our way alone, and there's a time in life when we would do well to reach out for help. I know there is a tendency to feel we might be shunned if we have an illness. Or maybe we just don't want to make the disease more real than it has to be by talking about it. We don't want to give it energy. But I'm not sure I would have handled the beginning stages of my diagnosis half as well as I did if I hadn't had the support of Howie, my brother and sister, my kids, and my friends. I also had an enormous advantage when I was connected to a wonderful woman I consider one of my early personal Sherpas.

Give yourself permission to accept help from a personal Sherpa.

I needed someone in my life who had been through breast cancer, someone who could guide and help me through it, someone who could talk me off the ledge when I was panicking. Someone very close to me connected me with the woman I'll call Sherpa Sherrie, and she was a big help in talking me down from the ledge of fear. Just knowing I could contact her if I was feeling crazed and scared was helpful. For me, the fear was actually the worst part.

On the night before my surgery, it was *her* voice and *her* words that I held on to because she was a real, living example that helped me trust that I was going to be intact when I awoke, and I wouldn't feel like I had been skinned alive.

Sherpa Sherrie also helped me with my other fears. She told me she wasn't that sick from chemo, only really tired sometimes. Her practical tip? She would plan her activities accordingly. She advised that I might want to take it easy during chemotherapy because I might be more tired than usual. For example, if she needed to go shopping with her daughter and go out to dinner with friends, Sherpa Sherrie would plan to do the shopping on one day and the dinner on another day.

As it turns out, I didn't feel tired most of the time. The intravenous cocktail I received to counteract the nausea during my infusions made me kind of wired the day after. Instead, I was somewhat tired the day after *that*. But in general, I felt pretty energetic. In general, I learned to accommodate the valleys.

Because of Sherpa Sherrie, whether or not I was tired, I wasn't lugging around the fear of getting chemotherapy. And that also included my fear of nausea. Sherpa Sherrie had not been nauseated. So despite the depiction of chemotherapy I saw on television and in movies, Sherpa Sherrie was a model for the fact that breast cancer chemotherapy does not make everyone violently ill.

I was going to have to get into the habit of talking to myself differently. I needed to write a new inner script.

The fear of infection also reared up. I was going to take the train in and out of New York City, and I was scared of exposure to trillions of germs being carried by the passengers in close quarters with me. Sherpa Sherrie told me that she was fine the whole time but advised me to be extra careful with some of my choices. She didn't ride the subway during chemo and went to the gym at off hours. I was careful, and I also got a shot that boosted my immune system considerably. The bottom line was that I never got sick or caught a cold during my chemo days. And I took the NYC train each time.

Sherpa Sherrie gave me fabulous, sound, practical advice for the night when I got home after surgery. She advised me to bring a loose-fitting button-down shirt. This would accommodate the four drains that would be coming out of my armpits because I was having a double mastectomy. I went shopping for a shirt that was pretty, one I wouldn't feel so bad about wearing. I ended up with a black-and-white checked button-down cotton shirt. I rolled up the sleeves, and it looked rather fashionable. I bought it in a big enough size so it wasn't tight on the bottom when I had four "bulbs" that were on the bottom of the leashes coming out of my pits.

Sherpa Sherrie found it extremely helpful to have an electric recliner chair to sleep in until the drains came out. That's because it's somewhat tricky to maneuver with the drains coming out of your armpits, especially if you have two coming out of each armpit from a double mastectomy. The chair would allow me to lie back and go to sleep without worrying about either Howie or me rolling over and tugging on the tubes. We borrowed a rather ugly reclining chair from my father-in-law—and it is still in my house. That first night I was never happier to see that ugly thing in my bedroom!

Sherpa Sherrie also warned me that one of the types of chemo might make my pee turn red. I totally forgot about this possibility. One day I made a princess pit stop after my chemo. I looked down and saw red in the porcelain throne and freaked. Synchronistically, Sherpa Sherrie called immediately after that "installment." I cried my heart out into the phone because I thought my red pee was a sure sign that I was dying. She reminded me it was the Red Devil or whatever the nickname is for that chemo. Whew! Was that all? Sheesh.

When I thought my Princess Diane von Brainisfried brain was actually becoming *totally* fried, Sherpa Sherrie told me about chemo brain. Guess what? It really is a thing. I thought I was losing my mind. I couldn't remember whether I brushed my teeth. I couldn't remember if I had eaten a piece of cake. I kept misplacing things the minute I put them down. Fortunately, I could laugh about it and started teasing myself. *Oh Romeo, Romeo, wherefore art my thingee dingee?*

Sherpa Sherrie was my earthly angel. But not all of my personal Sherpas were on the earth at the same time as me. My grandmother was another personal Sherpa who helped me through breast cancer.

As I mentioned earlier, my dad's mom, Lena Olian Young, was a source of strength. During my breast cancer journey, I drew on her spirit, courage, and strength, and I channeled her fortitude and practical nature. The night before my mastectomy surgery, I thought about Lena and invoked her motto: You do what you have to do. I felt her angel presence watching over me and encouraging me.

Personal Sherpas or no personal Sherpas, was the entire experience a cakewalk? That would be a no. I still had, and have, my struggles. But don't be shy about connecting to wise ones who have gone before you who know their way up the mountain. Give yourself permission to ask for their help. This help can make all the difference in how you experience a difficult situation.

Permission to Be Healthy

Giving yourself permission to be healthy is another important step toward a new, still-loving-your-life attitude. Take a baby step toward rewriting your own script by refusing to "own" breast cancer. How? My dear friend Nina told me not to say, "I have breast cancer." Instead say, "I've been diagnosed with breast cancer." Don't name it and don't claim it, and you'll start to reframe it. This will help you give yourself permission to be healthy by talking about a *diagnosis* and not talking about something that you *have*.

By talking about a diagnosis instead of allowing breast cancer to be like industrial grade glue stuck on you, the issue is merely loosely taped and easily washed off. It's not something you possess. It's not something you own. It's not something you have. It's not something with which you identify. You haven't even borrowed it. It's just passing through. If you have a cold, you don't identify with that. You are someone who is healthy who just happens to have a cold. In the same way, I was someone healthy who happened to be diagnosed with breast cancer. Even the docs described me as healthy—not even "otherwise healthy."

Giving myself permission to be healthy turned out to be a very important and powerful tool to help me get through with optimism and positivity. You see, if you're always telling yourself that you *have* cancer and feel like you own it, it can heartily inform your present worldview. The result can be that you are in illness default mode. Your illness might inform your waking days and sleeping nights. It might end up in your mind telling you that you are sick unless you question that presumption. No, I want you to default to the mindset that you are well, and if you feel sick, that's the aberration, and you'll deal with it.

This may not always be easy, and some people might really be struggling with their health in other areas. But giving yourself permission to be healthy and not owning breast cancer is something that can happen in your mind. It is not totally dependent on what is going on with your body. What you tell your mind to think can be something different than your current "reality."

Here's another key: To the extent that you can aim for the perspective that your default state is health, you will have another bullet in your ammunition belt for being mentally and emotionally sanguine. To the extent that I was able to achieve this outlook, a psychological burden was lifted off me that had been looming large when I was first diagnosed.

I encourage you to try your best to identify with health every single day. Make that your default expectation. If you don't feel well, you'll deal with that on a day-by-day basis. You're resilient, remember? You're healthy "in spite of." You're healthy . . . because. Just because.

Here's another perk. By giving myself permission to be a healthy person, I was more motivated and had more energy to do life's healthy dance—like eating healthily, exercising, and not giving up and dropping out of life's happiness roster. That's because every day didn't feel like a fight for mental survival. I defaulted to healthy thoughts and a healthy state of mind, which made what seemed like the mountain ahead something smaller than Mount Everest, even if it was bigger than a molehill.

Permission to Laugh

Laughter is truly the best medicine. If you don't believe me, I've got the Bible to back me up. "A merry heart doeth good like medicine, but a broken spirit drieth the bones." Proverbs 17:22 (KJV). Amen, princess sister.

As I said earlier, I've been told I laugh too much. Hey, I'm a princess, not the court jester, but we princesses need to laugh too. In fact, we have responsibilities the jester doesn't have, so laughter is even more important for us. And it just so happens that studies have not only shown that laughter fosters health and healing, it fosters better relationships, creativity, and problem solving. Who's laughing now?

Giving myself permission to be healthy turned out to be a very important and powerful tool to help me get through with optimism and positivity.

I first became aware of the healing benefits of laughter when I learned how Norman Cousins used laughter to help combat a serious, extremely painful, and life-threatening illness. He wrote about it in his book *Anatomy of an Illness*. Part of the regimen he decided to follow included binge watching funny movies. He discovered that laughter was an incredibly effective tool to help him deal with pain.10 He was not the only one to figure that out.

Researchers have begun to dig seriously into the issue of laughter and well-being. For example, when healthy adult volunteers in a research project at the University of Texas, Austin, watched a thirty-minute funny video, they had improvements in artery function and flexibility that lasted practically twenty-four hours. By contrast, the artery functionality decreased somewhat in the volunteers who watched a documentary. These University of Texas findings expanded upon another study at the University of Maryland Medical Center.[11] No worries, my royal friends. That doesn't mean documentaries will make you sick. It just means that if you think you're having a heart attack, after you call 911, watch The Three Stooges and not *An Inconvenient Truth*. Other studies also attribute many health benefits to laughter, such as strengthening your immune system, promoting better sleep, and relieving stress.[12]

You watch. Pretty soon, making someone laugh will be considered practicing medicine without a license! Giving yourself permission to be healthy aligns with the method of giving yourself permission to be happy. You are going to be healthy "in spite of" and challenging "who says." *I'm going to laugh in spite of breast cancer. Who says I can't laugh if I'm diagnosed with breast cancer?*

Giving myself permission to be happy included giving myself permission to laugh and use humor to make fun of what was going on, even when I was frightened. *Especially* when I was frightened. In challenging times, we often feel that humor isn't appropriate. You know what's not appropriate? Failing to survive mentally.

My dad's grandmother, Dena, whom he adored and whom I am named after, used to say, "As long as you can laugh." And that lady had her share of hardship as an immigrant who lost a son, Isidor (Izzy), in the Argonne forest in France during WWI, the day before Armistice Day.

Izzy Olian performed great acts of bravery and heroism for his men in the US Army, but the details are long lost, and the medal he was supposed to have received is lost in red tape and smoke. At any rate, that would not bring him back. Dena also lost a three-year-old daughter to a fever. Those hardships do not include the many other hardships of WWI, including losing countless friends and family in that war. But like my friend Fanny, she found a way to survive. And that way included laughter.

Of course, when you are in the thick of things and it feels like life has put a target on your head, it's not generally funny. But sometimes a target on your head is a good thing. It all depends on your perspective.

Many years ago, I heard about a restaurant designed for outdoor eating. When a patron sat down to eat, they were given a little paper hat to wear that had a bull's-eye on top of it. There were tons of pigeons in the vicinity. If you got lucky and a pigeon flying overhead crapped on your head, you got a free meal!

At one point during my treatment for breast cancer, I totally felt like there was a target with a bull's-eye on my head—but not the good kind with the paper hat. It was a breaking point. That sounds really bad, doesn't it? That sounds like you don't want to make fun of the situation, right? Wrong! The very thing that seemed to break me is actually funny to me now, whenever I look back on it with sober, dispassionate eyes.

As I said earlier in my princess-takes-on-cancer story, I went through two lumpectomies, then soldiered on through a double mastectomy. Then there was reconstruction, which started as Pancakesville on my chest and gradually expanded with the expanders that felt like rocks on my chest. Then came chemotherapy. I was totally bald for a long time. But even that didn't send me like a screaming banshee up and over a cliff. I never really had a good palace pop-up pity party, freak out, or big three-ring circus cry—until one event got me totally wigged out.

It was the itty-bitty tiny tattoos. Yep, you heard me right. The itty-bitty tiny tattoos. The docs needed the technicians to place small dots to mark where the radiation would be aimed each time. They were essentially using my body as a map. They used permanent tattoo ink when they did the first round of mapping so they would know where to mark thereafter without having to do the mapping again. Most of the dots were almost imperceptible, but one set of double dots, which looked like a quotation mark, went right between my newly reconstructed, perfect and perky "girls" in that beautiful spot known as the décolleté. That was my breaking point!

I cried and cried. I remembered about the little restaurant with the paper hats and the pigeons taking a bull's-eye crap on people's heads, and this is what I thought: *Where's my free meal? Can you hear me up there? Where's my free meal?*

Yep, it's true. Even in the midst of cancer-treatment-induced breakdown, my mind connected the thing that was freaking me out to something funny. You can take the princess out of the fun house, but apparently, you can't take the fun house out of the princess.

Permission Granted

If you're struggling with the idea of giving yourself permission to be healthy and happy, then I, Princess Diane von Brainisfried, grant you that permission now. I am a princess, after all. Consider it done. Permission granted.

But it's really better if you give *yourself* permission. Even in the face of serious health challenges, remember to claim your right to a good life. And remember to laugh.

Don't be shy about connecting to wise ones who have gone before you who know their way up the mountain.

11

Humor Is Everywhere

*Allowing yourself to find the funny helps you feel optimistic
because you learn the edges of your own ability to
take what comes and take it as it comes.*
–Princess Diane von Brainisfried

If you're in the middle of a palace pop-up pity party, it can be hard to find the humor in things. But actually, humor is everywhere. Really. I mean, isn't the very idea of a palace pop-up pity party funny? I was even able to find some humor after my father's death. No doubt, I was channeling his grandmother Dena and her "as long as you can laugh" mindset.

After my dad passed, my sibs and I had to select his coffin. In the Jewish religion, it's traditional to be buried in a plain pine box. As a matter of fact, it's basically a mitzvah to order a plain pine box so the worms can get at it faster. Dust to dust and all that rot. Pardon the pun. I might not have the rationale right, but the fact of the plain pine box I'm clear on.

At the gravesite, as my dad's coffin was being lowered into the earth, I had a crazy mishmash of thoughts. *How long does it take before bones are dust?* I remembered speculation about how long it took a Styrofoam cup to decompose, and then I thought about my implants,

*The Lord giveth,
and the Lord then taketh
away, but sometimes the
surgeons giveth back.*

which were essentially plastic. I realized that when it was my turn in the ground, two plastic mounds would be left after the rest of me had turned to dust. That image made me laugh.

But I was already in a humor-friendly frame of mind before I even got to the grave-site. After giving the eulogy at the funeral, I left to find the ladies room. During my dogged search, I glanced up over a door and saw the sign of relief that read "Restroom." A thought crossed my mind that I immediately attributed to my dad: I'm sure glad it doesn't say *eternal* rest room!

My dad would have been sooo proud of me for that funny thought. And I sooo wanted to be able to tell him, but on a gut level, I felt clearly, powerfully, and energetically sure that Dad was the source of the thought, so I didn't need to tell him. Dad would have loved that I was still able to smile and laugh during his funeral. My dad had been all about humor. And seriously, what parent wants their kid to suffer? I knew he was laughing with me.

How did being able to see the funny stuff in a sad situation make me feel? Resilient. Strong. Survivor-blessed. Allowing yourself to find the funny helps you feel optimistic because you learn the edges of your own ability to take what comes and take it as it comes.

And I needed to find optimism during my cancer journey, I needed chuckle-berry stew to chew on. When I came home from my mastectomy, I had expanders inserted under my chest wall. They were essentially thick plastic bags with a port through which they could be blown up—expanded—little by little. Every two weeks or so, a liquid solution was infused through the port. If you can imagine filling a balloon with liquid instead of air, that was what it was like. The purpose of the expanders was to stretch my skin so a saline or silicone implant could eventually be inserted. And voilà, two new beautiful breasts.

In addition to the ports for the expanders on either side of my chest, I had another port in my chest wall where the pic line was to be inserted each time I received chemotherapy. This prevented my arms from looking like a voodoo doll with a serious curse problem. But that made a total of three ports that I was walking around with. One day, a funny thought came to my mind: I had more ports than a horny sailor!

The chemo itself was hazmat worthy, and I have proof. Some patients referred to it as Red Devil Chemo. What could be funny about that? Nothing, until I thought about what was happening. The nurses came into the room and started gowning up in what were essentially hazmat suits: long gowns, gloves, masks, and booties. I thought they were preparing for surgery, not a simple infusion. I asked them why they were cloaking themselves in gear that appeared suitable for protecting them from a villainous gas attack. Meanwhile, did I have a gown on or any other protection? No. Zip. Nadda. I got nothin'. One of the nurses explained that the reason they were taking such precautions was because the chemo was so toxic, getting even the tiniest drip on their bare skin would be as catastrophic as a bad burn. It would be as if fire had touched their skin, and they would immediately have to go to the emergency room. Maybe even get a skin graft.

When I heard this, my mind was like a pinball caroming off of the walls of a pinball machine. *Is that so? You mean to tell me the stuff is so toxic that it could cause a serious burn? And not only am I not protected and gowned up, but you are shoving that stuff into my veins! Well, golly gee, that doesn't seem fair.* But even though it was scary to think of it that way, it was so ironic that it was downright funny.

Chemo, even chemo that is not necessarily as toxic as Red Devil Chemo, can have some pretty problematic side effects. One type of chemo caused what I called "the Phoebe, paella, and maestro incident." The side effects of a certain type of chemo I received could mess with my fingernails and toenails by either causing them to turn black or promoting infection. I had the honor of receiving both indignities, but only to my two big toes.

The nurses give patients ice packs to pack your fingers and toes in during the infusions of this type of chemo. For some reason, my two big toes decided to rebel and became infected. Later, the nails actually fell off. Later still, another breast cancer survivor suggested I do what she does: stop getting pedicures and go to a podiatrist. I started doing this, and it made a huge difference.

Infected toes hurt. A lot. They hurt partly because the nails had lifted, so anytime something wiggled them, like a shoe rubbing or the bed sheets at night, the pain would ring loud and clear. I couldn't seem to clear it up. With chemo, it can be tough to shake an infection, and this infection went on and on, all summer long. I couldn't wear closed-toe shoes because the pressure from the top of a closed-toe shoe would have been excruciating. Luckily, it was summer, and I could wear sandals everywhere I went.

What happens sometimes when there's an infection? Ooze. Which is different from ouzo, a fantastic Greek aperitif. Both will momentarily become relevant. Regarding my ill-fated, tender toes, I was pretty good at hiding them with bandages. And it didn't look gross or anything. It just hurt. Luckily, the secret was between me and my doctor. Nobody ever noticed. That is, nobody except and until Phoebe.

One summer's night, Howie and I were invited to a paella dinner given by a "fremily" of ours (friends who are like family) consisting of the Greek maestro, his wife, a renowned musician, and a few other people. The maestro is a famous conductor whose paella dinners are legendary. Thankfully, it was a hot summer night, as the rock singer Meatloaf would say, so my sandals would not make anyone notice that something odd was afoot.

Howie and I walked in the door, a happy hug fest ensued, and then (insert Jaws movie music here) Phoebe—the family's large, loveable, harmless, mixed breed dog—entered. Okay, Phoebe is a mutt. But

Phoebe's harmless rating was upgraded to usually harmless. That night, Phoebe was on a reconnaissance mission. Her eyes were wild, her head was down, and what she was aiming at was clear: my infected toes in my open-toe sandals. Catnip for a dog!

Now we princesses who have reached "lady" status are pretty astute. Who among us hasn't had to fend off a sniffing mutt or two when out for a walk on the palace grounds when it's that time of month? This how-to stuff has been passed down from queens to daughters for centuries. Palace rumors tell that Queen Victoria even had a special muzzle for hyper-interested curs—oh, wait . . . that was for her husband.

But what did I know about a chemo-compromised toe and a dog's desires? I soon learned. Phoebe was relentlessly trying to lift my infected big toenail! I used to think that the method of torture we've all heard about, putting bamboo shoots under fingernails of prisoners, was apocryphal. Now I know it's a real thing. And it hurts!

And so that otherwise magical night's intrigue began. Phoebe sent me hopping and twirling trying to get her off me. I don't think anyone noticed, but if they did, they probably just thought I was dog-skittish. When we sat down to dinner for the luscious meal, things really got sticky. Phoebe made a beeline for my toes under the table. She knew I was trapped, the clever girl! She had me right where she wanted me.

That's when the dinner party *really* started—Phoebe's dinner party. The beast began licking my toes. Up under and over, lifting and sniffing my poor little nail that was hanging on for dear life. I held my leg up. Phoebe followed. I twirled my leg. Phoebe followed. Was it painful? Let's put it this way: Even if it had been a cloudy, rainy night, I still would have seen stars.

Luckily, my dear hostess saw me squirming, but being a gracious hostess, she asked no questions. She got Phoebe out from her spot and me out of my dilemma. I'll tell ya. Whatever I did wrong in my last lifetime, karma's a bitch. Literally.

How did being able to see the funny stuff in a sad situation make me feel? Resilient. Strong. Survivor-blessed.

From head to toe, my cancer experience had its funny moments. When I first had my head shaved and was getting my wig on, along with my groove back, the wig purveyor instructed me on the ways of putting on a wig. I was a little intimidated. If you wear contact lenses, you might be able to relate. When you were trying to put in your first pair, did you get the feeling that out of all the contact wearers in the world, you would be the only one to have the distinct honor of not being able to get them in your eyes? I felt that way about contacts, and I felt that way about the wig. It was a long, thick forest of a prosthesis, and it was intimidating to my head.

I didn't really get a chance to practice at the wig shop because the guy handed it to me and guided it onto my head. But any of you who have tried to work the television, remote, or cable, know you don't just read the instructions once and know how to watch what you want. There's a period of frustration and forgetting before it becomes rote. That's what it was like with my wig. I had a period of frustration and forgetting how to put it on.

The day after I had my head shaved was the day I was on my own. Cold turkey. I woke up, brushed my teeth, took a shower, and pulled my new furry friend out of the box. I was still a little intimidated. *Princess, it doesn't bite, and it's not rocket science,* I said to myself. I shook the big rat to fluff it up. Then I bent over to make it easier to pull the elastic part onto my head without the long strands of hair getting in the way. I managed to wiggle it on with a bit of twisting and turning—except, when I stood up and shook my head from side to side to settle the wig in, I couldn't see anything! Talk about not being able to see the forest for the trees.

You know those cartoons where explorers are walking through a dense forest and they part a thick bushy growth of leaves so they can continue walking? That's what it felt like. I couldn't find anywhere that resembled a part for the side bang. I was looking straight ahead through a dense forest of hair.

Then the tears started showing up. I was scared that I was going to have to stay bald because I wouldn't be able to figure out how to wear wigs. I shuffled it and flipped one strand of hair over the other, desperately trying to figure out how to make the bushy animal sit on my head properly. The thing completely covered the front of my face. I parted the strands that hung down in front of my eyes and looked in the mirror. Staring back at me was a dead ringer for Snuffleupagus. What was I gonna do?

Then it dawned on me that I might have the thing on backwards. I did! I pulled the beast off, whipped it around, and pulled it on properly.

That story alone was worth the price of admission. And it was certainly worth the email I got from my dad—one of the last emails my dad wrote to me before he passed.

Dear Dee,

Forward (or backward), the new haircut looks spectacular. Wear it in good health and secure in the knowledge that little by little, it is being supplanted by your own crop that is silently waiting to dispossess this intruder. Hair or no hair, you are still the same ebullient, cheerful, lusty, delightful good soul who is an expert at turning lemons into delicious lemonade or even lemon chiffon pie and then sharing it with everyone around.

With all our love and admiration—Dad and Mom

My dad wasn't the only one who had something to say about my head. A friend of mine came to visit after my double mastectomy surgery when I was flat as a flounder frittata because reconstruction wasn't visibly underway. She had only love in her heart and was trying to make me feel better, but my shiny head was a shoo-in for an Elmer Fudd stunt double. "Well, you know, I can still tell by your face that you're not a boy!" she said. Flat chest, shiny head, and *still* she could tell I was a girl!

As Queen Victoria famously said, "Well, butter my butt and call me a biscuit!"

Well, maybe somebody else said that, but the truth is, humor fosters optimism and a healthy psyche, even if it's at your own expense. Because let's face it, the whole damn thing is at your own expense! Humor promotes resilience too, which is a sharp tool in the optimist's bag of tricks. Besides, if you can laugh at it, the whole situation bites less. When my dad told me that my mastectomy was really only about removing two large moles, it helped me enormously. It downplayed the seriousness of the ordeal. And you sure as hell have to figure out where to put your mind the night before a mastectomy. My dad's comment, coupled with my brother's statement that I was going to get a new pair of Park Avenue boobs, were mind-saving bits of humor the night before my mastectomy. And *my* new Park Avenue boobs were going to be paid by insurance. Talk about perspective!

Sometimes you have to take the humor up to a whole nuther level. I decided to go for broke. On the day of my surgery I was scared, but whistling in the dark made it easier. My form of whistling was laughing and singing. As I was wheeled into the operating room, the docs and I had our own little musical going. I started it off, and the doctors and nurses were real pals about joining in. Hit it now (and sung to the tune of "Bye Bye Birdie"):

Bye-bye boobies,
I'm gonna miss you so,
Why'd ya have to go?
Bye-bye boobies,
Bye-bye boobies,

Ta-ta, oh sweetie pies.
Bye-bye boobies,
Time for you to fly,
Hope that I don't die,
Time to say good-bye.

My surgery took place in the early spring, right before Easter and Passover. My room had a huge picture window with an absolutely gorgeous and glam view of New York City. There were floor to ceiling windows and a huge panorama of twinkling city lights. At least *that* was a perk. When I woke up from the surgery, I had two long, leash-like tubes hanging out of each armpit. My first thought: *Who let the dogs out?* The drains are *not* the most fun scene from *Mastectomy: The Musical.*

After one night, they send you home. Howie had stayed overnight in the room with me, thank goodness, because I really needed the support. We left before breakfast, and when we got home, it was still breakfast time. We were both hungry. Howie was trying his best to be helpful. He wanted to make breakfast for us, and he was pondering what to make. He took one look at me and said, "Anyone for pancakes?"

Nice. I laughed and thought it was funny, and it was. But that didn't mean it was easy. It wasn't easy. I didn't fool myself, and I don't want to fool you. It's not easy, but we don't have to make it harder on ourselves than we need to. That's why we've got to find the funny. Thank the Lord I gave myself permission to find the funny.

The Lord giveth, and the Lord then taketh away, but sometimes the surgeons giveth back. My whole adult life, I had been the gal with the big boobs who had to wear the serviceable, no-nonsense, nurse shoe kind of bra. When I came out of surgery, hiding beneath bandages where two big cantaloupes used to be were two little Easter egg ta-tas. Can you imagine? I loved my plastic surgeon. He was the best of the best. It was Easter and Passover. Had he been Jewish, maybe instead of Easter eggs, he would have given me big, ta-ta matzo balls.

I tell you this to provide the full impact of how I felt so you can understand my initial dismay. I like to make this analogy for the boyz. If you were swinging a nine-inch shlong around, dazzling the ladies with your lasso, and then one day someone chopped it down to three inches, I would imagine you'd need a period of identity adjustment too.

I might have been a tad happier with the body evolution if I had gotten a tummy tuck along with the deal. But the doc who evaluated me for that said that there wasn't enough stomach tissue to be able to reconstruct a set of knockers with which I would be happy. This was just one more example of how bad news was also good news. Yay! I couldn't get a tummy tuck at the same time because I didn't have enough tummy to tuck.

Here's the irony. They say that man plans and God laughs. A few years earlier, I had a chance to have a tummy tuck when I had a hysterectomy and was the owner of two C-section scars. I opted not to get a tummy tuck because my mother was afraid for me to be under anesthesia any longer than I had to be and my sister discovered that if, God forbid, I should get breast cancer, one place they harvest skin for reconstruction is your tummy. We all came to the consensus to leave well enough alone, and I said no-go to the flatten-my-tummy show.

Should I have kicked myself later? That would have been Monday morning quarterbacking. Besides, if I were perfect, people might hate me.

Reconstruction had numerous funny moments. There is nothing like defining your breast size by the number of ccs added through the expander ports. How big was I? Another 500ccs. When I was "fully expanded" and had implant surgery, the day came to remove the gauze pads and have a look. I was astonished. Knock, knock. Excuse me? Excuse me? Doctor? Doctor? I don't mean to be a pain, but did you forget something in the operating room? Check your pockets maybe. *You seem to have misplaced my nipples!*

Turns out that is part of the deal. They take all the insides and part of the outside too! If I wanted nipples put back, I was going to have to go to the nipple store. As it turned out, there was a sort of a nipple store. You could either have another surgery down the road to give you mock nipples made of skin taken from your groin area or you could actually get 3D nipple tattoos! At least I had options. I

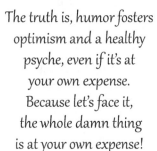

The truth is, humor fosters optimism and a healthy psyche, even if it's at your own expense. Because let's face it, the whole damn thing is at your own expense!

elected the 3D tattoos. I had mine crafted by an amazingly talented woman. Rumor had it that she had done the Sistine Chapel—in another life.

Among the many issues I had to deal with during my breast cancer journey, a big one was handling the new me resulting from the physical changes to my body. I had a lot of things to figure out. Who was Princess Diane von Brainisfried now that her physical appearance had been so dramatically altered?

My brother tried to talk some sense into me. "You are not your boobs. I'd hate to think people relate to you that way. Pretty shallow."

I was grateful, and I heard him, but I found myself contemplating the fact that I knew plenty of people who didn't swim in the deep end. Heck, many people didn't even know how to swim. I had to make a shift, an adjustment in terms of how I thought about myself physically. I put a positive spin on my new figure: new and improved. I looked at my new "peaks" as perks. They were youthful, perky. They were stargazers. And I figured that change could be a good thing if I let it.

The point was that life can hand you some doozies to deal with and whoopers to wrestle with. When that happens, you've got two choices and two choices only: You either take it on the chin or you'll take it up the arse.

Comedian Jerry Lewis talked about how he witnessed the healing power of laughter firsthand. He had just finished a show when one of his people informed him that there was a lady outside who was absolutely sobbing. She said she had to see Jerry. When they met, she said, "I need a hug." He hugged her and told her that if they hugged any harder, he'd have to get a room.

The reason for the woman's visit was a powerful tribute to the healing power of humor. She told Jerry that she had not laughed in seven years, but that night, Jerry had made her laugh. Her son had been killed in Saigon, and she had not been able to get over her sorrow. But that night, when Jerry had made her laugh, she felt she could get on with her life and learn to deal with it.

When you can laugh through pain, you realize that you've come back from the deep beyond, that it's possible to live again. You realize that your resilience is reliably honed. You're like a deep-sea diver coming up from the deep, and the bubbles have come out of your blood.

Years before my mastectomy, I felt terribly blue for months after my first miscarriage. I just couldn't shake the awesomely horrible depression. One day, when I was at the gym, something struck me as funny, and the waters of darkness parted. I was in the ladies' shower area. The showers were individual stalls, and the shower stall doors went almost all the way down, but not completely. I saw a woman's feet below the shower stall doors, and for some crazy reason, seeing just her feet sticking out at the bottom of the door struck me as hysterical. I laughed aloud uncontrollably, and then I felt complete relief. I was back.

Laughter can do that. It can help you get on with your life. That is why I kept making jokes even when I was facing my double mastectomy. It was my way of drawing on the tools of resilience in my treasure chest. I used humor as my armor to get me through. It worked.

Some friends have told me—almost as an admonishment—that when I laugh in the face of challenges, I am laughing out of nervousness. My answer to that is this: Who cares? To the extent that it keeps me from crying, I *am* really laughing. And . . . don't look a gift horse in the mouth.

Allowing yourself to find the funny helps you feel optimistic because you learn the edges of your own ability to take what comes and take it as it comes.

12

Simple Princess Positivity Pointers for Pulling Out of a Funk

Become a word chiropractor and make an attitude adjustment.
–Princess Diane von Brainisfried

*E*veryone needs a little boost on the days when we are down in the dumpster. Add the pressures, fears, and worries of breast cancer to everyday concerns and you've got a recipe for some serious stress. Whenever I felt the blues overtake me or I became frenetic over one thing or other—like wondering whether I was going to die from breast cancer—I would try to remember some sage words someone had said (and sometimes that someone was me), and it would calm me and help me to gain perspective. There's a lot to be said for that. Sometimes those words were as warm and comforting as a steaming bowl of oatmeal on a winter's morning. But I needed both words of wisdom and practices to keep me chill in the chill.

I stored some of my favorite princess positivity practices in my palace treasure chest, and I'm going to share a few of them with you. Some of them are from my own tiara-topped head. Some of them are known aphorisms that you have probably heard. Hey, if it ain't broke, don't break it!

Good Old-Fashioned Perspective

I may have been born with what Fanny called "a sunny disposition," but that's not to say that I'm immune to bouts of the blues. I have found that one of the best antidotes to the blues and to the creeping claws of fear is good old-fashioned perspective. Perspective rules!

From time to time when I felt sorry for myself, I would recall how my dad used to cite a well-known saying: There once was a man who felt sorry for himself because he had no shoes. Then he met a man who had no feet. The image of the man with no feet in contrast to merely having no shoes is a sobering thought. It is a good way to shift your thinking and to contemplate the relative nature of hardship. Some people can have a major meltdown when a manicured nail gets chipped. You might imagine how this phrase would be a useful tool to get a grip. It helped me get a grip many times when much more than a broken nail was bothering me.

Here are a few more wise sayings my dad taught me over the years that came in really handy-dandy to gain perspective:

Into every life a little rain must fall.

This too shall pass.

It's all a matter of mind over matter; I don't mind, and it don't matter.

I used these sayings over and over again to help me through the breast cancer journey.

My sibs and I heard another of my dad's favorites so often when we called to ask how he was doing that we decided to engrave it on his headstone, along with the "in loving memory" and birth/death information: *If it doesn't get any worse, I won't complain about it not being any better.* Headstone-worthy, I'd say. I can hear him laughing about it. I'm sure we would have his heartfelt approval.

Fanny had a wonderful French expression that means (loosely and not literally) "you are making a mountain out of a molehill." It's perfect for you Francophile princesses out there. The phrase is, *Tu churches midi à quatorze heures.* Literally, it means "You're looking for noon at 4:00." I don't know how they get to the mountain and molehill interpretation, but that's what it means, and it's a good one. It was applicable when I became overwhelmed by having to keep track of the many doctor appointments or I was fretting over (okay, another admission) a broken nail. But I didn't have a nail file on me! I know you get it.

Remember, too, the wise words of my yoga teacher, which are spot-on for keeping perspective: It's not what is happening to you that's important, it's what you *tell* yourself is happening to you that's important. Truly, there is more than one way to look at life's ups and downs. And a positive perspective can move you from of a sense of helplessness into a place of personal power.

Knowing that it's what you tell yourself that is the important thing reminds you that *you* get to choose how you look at a situation, how you interpret it. For example, here's another phrase that I frequently invoke: If it's a rainy, dreary day, maybe that's how it looks to some people. Yes, I could see it as a rainy, dreary day. But does that help my spirits? Nope. This is how I call it on a rainy and dreary day. I tell myself it's a cozy, ducky day. Or as an homage to my opera background, a "cosi fan duckie" day.

The word *cozy* changes everything. Do you see the power of that? Rainy and dreary versus cozy and ducky. Cozy gives me power. Cozy makes me feel good. Cozy makes me feel... cozy. Cozy doesn't make me feel helpless against the elements. Cozy isn't battleship gray. Cozy is pink. Cozy is creamy. Cozy is hot chocolate. Cozy is a cup of tea with honey.

In the movie *Parenthood*, there is a great scene in which Steve Martin's character is worrying and fretting about life being messy and the fact that there are no guarantees about anything. Enter the wise grandmother. She's got a big, knowing smile, and she talks about how she took a ride on a roller coaster when she was nineteen. She couldn't believe how a ride could make her so frightened, scared, sick, excited, and thrilled—all at the same time. She talks of other people who only had the nerve to go on the merry-go-round. She turned her nose

Perspective is the number one priority in my hierarchy of thoughts to beat the breast cancer blues.

up at those people. The merry-go-round just goes around. It's got nothing else to offer. No, Grandma liked the roller coaster! She felt that you squeezed so much more out of life when you got on that thing. It was more exciting precisely because it went up and down. She didn't like the boring safety of the merry-go-round.

Way to go, Grandma! That's certainly a fresh perspective on the ups and downs of life. Her worldview illustrates that there are different ways to look at the travails that befall us. It's part of the cycle, and some people feel that it is invigorating.

This following princess positivity practice is a quintessential perspective tool that you simply must keep at the ready. It saved me many times during my cancer journey. I don't know how I pulled this gem out of my tiara, but it's a winner-winner-lobster-dinner. I call it the yeahbut practice. Here's how it's used. Let's say your inner mind starts to complain about the fact that you are facing a long road of chemotherapy. If your mind goes, *wahhh, wahhh, wahhh,* here's what you do. Tell yourself, *Yeahbut, yeahbut, yeahbut . . . yeah, but I get to live.*

I used this strategy to help gain perspective (and a grip) *continuously* throughout my cancer journey. It was, and still is, my biggest go-to princess positivity practice for perspective. I still use it when I start to obsess or stress about the residual effects of my cancer treatment. As a matter of fact, I use it so much that if the expression were shoes, I would have worn through ten pairs by now.

Here's another example of how to use the yeahbut strategy. Let's say it's hotter than Hades outside in the grimy city, and you feel yuckity-yuck-muckity. You're feeling sorry for yourself because you're hot and hairless, stuck wearing a wig that's making you sweat like nobody's business. You feel the inner whiner bubbling up to the surface of your mind, but you smile instead. You have a strategy, so fahgheddaboudit! You dig into your treasure chest of positivity strategies and tell yourself, *Yeahbut, yeahbut, yeahbut . . . yeah, but I get to live!* The great thing about yeahbut yeahbut yeahbut is that it not only brings perspective, it stokes your sense of humor at the same time. And humor is the A+ resilience strategy.

What happens if you find yourself already wallowing in a full-blown palace pop-up pity party—the kind with paper hats, streamers, blowy horns, layer cake, candles, pin the tail on the donkey, the whole nine yards? You are in that space with both feet firmly planted and no clue how to talk yourself off the ledge. How do you get out of there?

Here's a solution I learned from a brilliant physician friend of mine. I call it the "cows in a line going home" strategy. When cows go from the field to the barn, they walk in a line, asses to noses. One by one, they follow each other in a single file toward their destination. One after the other—maybe hundreds of them—ass to nose, ass to nose. What if one of them didn't want to go to the barn? What if she wanted to break free? What if she thinks she's stuck in a big line of behinds and noses? She has no chains on her. She has no leash. All she has to do is turn around and walk the other way.

Likewise, all we have to do if we are going in a direction we don't like is turn around and walk the other way. We aren't stuck continuing on the path we are on. We might think we are, but we aren't. Maybe I haven't remembered the farming principles exactly right, but the metaphor is quite mooving. So say to your palace pop-up pity party, "I'm turning around, and I am so outta here!"

Perspective is the number one priority in my hierarchy of thoughts to beat the breast cancer blues. Having a few of these sayings that you can keep in your pocket, ready to pull out when a challenge arises, is a stellar idea. It's like checking out the emergency exits on an airplane before the flight or in a theater before a movie. You want to know these things ahead of time because sometimes it's hard to think clearly in an emergency. These strategies have your back, and you will always be prepared.

Don't Borrow Trouble

Abandon needless pregame worrying. The truth is, things aren't always as bad as they seem, so don't borrow trouble.

Here's how I applied this on my cancer journey.

I have never been a fan of barfing. As a matter of fact, it is one of my biggest fears in life, along with its precursor, being nauseated. When my oldest son had a virus that brought on his first experience with vomiting at about age five and didn't cry, I was awestruck. I couldn't believe that this little boy handled with relative nonchalance what I considered a traumatic incident. I knew that if I had been the one bent over the porcelain throne, I would have been bawling my eyes out while simultaneously retching, which perhaps in itself is pretty awe-inspiring. Being able to do both at once, that is. When I realized that chemotherapy was a pretty inescapable option, my mind began a campaign of FOTU (Fear Of Throwing Up). Everything about chemo seemed to have throwing up in the vicinity. I wasn't merely borrowing trouble, I was stealing it.

I wasted a lot of energy and expended too much stress on these fears because I pretty much escaped nausea, and I never threw up from my treatments. The medical community has made great strides in counteracting these undesirable side effects. Yes, some people really do have a hard time with the chemo and treatments. But the point is, what I thought was absolute and inescapable—a wretched next few months of my life lived in nausea and retching—never happened. And most of the time, I actually felt pretty great. Don't borrow trouble.

I also worried about pain from the two lumpectomies and double mastectomy. Yes, I am sure that there is a spectrum of how people fare post-surgery when it comes to pain. But on the whole, it was pretty uneventful for me in terms of pain. Again, modern medicine has come a long way.

Another sinkhole I was worried about was lymphedema, a swelling that can occur due to lymph node removal. The swelling can be pretty darn severe. To date, I have not suffered from it. Fingers crossed. I have to be careful not to have my blood pressure taken or receive shots in my left arm, which is the side on which my lymph nodes were removed. I have to be careful to avoid cutting myself on my left hand or arm and to be vigilant about not getting infections. So this is what I tell myself: I'm careful. That's about all I *can* do. Don't borrow trouble.

I was also worried I wouldn't have full range of motion with my arms. I did the exercises they gave me. So far, so good. I've got my full range of motion back.

And then there were the perceived perils of estrogen therapy. While I was absolutely grateful that I was estrogen-receptive and therefore a candidate for hormone therapy in the form of estrogen blocker pills, I was extremely anxious about what this would mean to my body and skin. The pills were going to block every bit of estrogen in my body. Would I start to shrivel up like a prune or grow hair in unseemly places? Was femininity totally going to be reamed out of me? The worry and fear were real.

It didn't help that one of my doctors told me he had seen havoc wreaked on his patients' skin because of these pills. That statement alone from a respected figure put me in palace pop-up pity party mode and prompted an immediate call to one of my besties. I went all boo-hooing about what I was *sure* was imminently going to happen to me.

Of course, my friend calmed me down, reminding me that so many of the fears I harbored were things I thought were going to happen that never happened. She reminded me of the many times I had worried needlessly. Apart from worrying about nausea and vomiting that never materialized, I had also worried that the steroids I was on during the therapy would make me fat. They never made me fat. I had heard that you become massively tired from chemo, and I was worried about that. That didn't happen either. There were one or two days during the cycle when I was a bit more tired than usual, but that was it. I was worried about my teeth going bad, and I was worried about getting a big infection and dying from it. Neither of those things happened.

The lesson: Dump the pregame worrying. If something comes your way that needs to be addressed and you start to worry, the good news is, you will have learned many excellent and effective strategies to help you handle it. And what was one of those strategies my father and his mother taught us? We'll do what has to be done.

In the School of Practical Philosophy, I learned that we have to train our minds like we train a puppy. We wouldn't let a puppy run wild in the house and crap all over the carpet, would we? Well, okay . . . mine does. Sometimes. But I don't like it, and I tell her that. We can't let our mind wander wherever it wants to and crap all over *us* either. We have to train it. In philosophy class, we learn to help our minds behave with practical wisdom, and later, in the more advanced classes, we include daily meditation.

My dear royal friends, you are learning to train your mind through all of these strategies that help you reboot, refocus, and revitalize.

And don't borrow trouble.

Watch Your Mouth!

The following idea is going to rock your breast cancer craziness off its rocker. As soon as someone you know (and that someone might be you) has a diagnosis of breast cancer or any other tough medical challenge, here's what you do: You make the next leap on the ladder to happiness by calling it an adventure.

Earlier, I suggested that you substitute the word *challenge* for the word *problem* because doing so is liberating and empowering. Likewise, looking at a challenging situation as an adventure as opposed to a problem is a powerful way to find inner strength. Of course, what we are really doing is reframing the situation into something positive.

As I also mentioned earlier, I learned to look at problems as challenges when I was working as an attorney. I'd like to expand on that story now because this lesson had a life-changing impact on my thinking and psyche. I had a veritable pyramid of bosses in that world. There were bosses, chief bosses, and at the top of the pyramid, the Chief. One day, the Chief came into my poor-excuse-for-an-office cubicle and casually asked me to handle a certain critically important, high visibility legal issue and get back to him as soon as possible.

I had no idea why he skipped over the chief bosses and bosses— the attorneys who had actual doors on their offices—to bring the issue to me. Maybe it was a test to see how I handled pressure. Maybe he was trying to do me in. Maybe he was trying to help me shine.

I can't remember what this critically important, high profile issue was, I just remember the fear. I was as scared as a chicken in a barnyard of foxes. To make matters worse, right before he waltzed into my cubicle, I had just eaten—actually, basically inhaled—a box of sticky, jellied fruit-flavored candies. Some of them, including the black ones, were so tenaciously stuck in and on my teeth that I couldn't open my mouth and talk. All I could do was nod and agree with everything he said—which included accepting the project.

Not only was I already on overload and swamped with work, I had absolutely no idea how to solve the issue he had just handed off to me. And not only did I have no idea where to start, I had no idea what category the problem fit into. Was it fish or fowl? Reptile or amphibian? I had no prior knowledge of that area of the law. I was stalled, stumped, and stymied.

The one thing I did know was that when the Chief handed me a problem, I could not hand it back to him with a note saying I didn't know how to solve it. If I couldn't solve the Chief's problem, I was not even worth one of the legal pads the office ordered in discounted bulk.

Why didn't I ask another attorney at the firm for help? I might have been ignorant about the problem, but I was no fool. Going to another attorney would have been like serving a bleeding fish to a school of sharks. That was not going to happen. After my initial panic, I realized that the only thing to do was to figure it out on my own.

And then a miracle happened. My inner voice whispered to me, *Don't call this a problem, call it a challenge.* And as soon as I characterized the task as a challenge and not a problem, inspiration hit. Something shifted in my mind. It felt like the top lifted off my head and something physical was done to my brain. Suddenly, the project seemed friendly, something I wanted to work on as opposed to run away from. By calling the task a challenge instead of a problem, the energy in my brain and soul shifted from something negative to something positive.

Henry J. Kaiser once said that problems are only opportunities in work clothes. I say they wear party dresses and ball gowns! What happens when we face a challenge? We rise to it. On the other hand, when we face a problem, we sink a little. When I used the word *challenge*, I felt like I had let the sun in and shed some light on what I needed to do. And gosh darn it, it wasn't long before I had figured it all out.

This lesson stayed with me. When I characterized an issue as a problem, it was exactly that—a problem. And I couldn't figure out what to do. But when I characterized the same thing as a challenge, something inside me changed, and I figured it out.

You might remember another fabulous strategy I talked about earlier, one I picked up from my friend Nina: Say you have been *diagnosed* with cancer, not that you *have* cancer. Can you hear and feel the difference? Don't own the cancer. Don't make it something that is yours, as if it were a part of your essence or being. Don't name it and claim it. Please think to yourself, *I'll have none of that.*

What fabulous advice, *n'est-ce pas?* I had to catch myself a thousand times before I remembered to do this. And I still occasionally lapse. I'm still learning and growing. If I accidentally trip up and say, "I have breast cancer," I immediately rephrase the sentence to "I was diagnosed with breast cancer." Making the change from an ownership to a diagnosis changes the energy of the beast in my mind. It's something that doesn't grip me. It's apart from me instead of a part of me. It's something I can deal with, something from which I have some distance, something that is not a part of me like my foot, my eyes, or my tiara. And yes, I certainly do have a tiara.

Using this strategy of watching my words and not claiming ownership over cancer was a brilliant strategy for me. It was instrumental in helping me to continue to *feel* healthy and give myself permission to *label* myself healthy.

Another example of reframing happened when I did some vigorous activity with my wig on and felt uncomfortably sticky from the heat. That happened a lot when I walked through Central Park in the dog days of August for my doctor appointments. So I reframed what was happening to me. A princess doesn't sweat, she mists. As long as I was misting and not sweating, I could handle the *shvitz.*

It's so important that you understand how much power the words you use have, and that includes the words in your thoughts. It is truly imperative that you understand this concept so you can manage your words and use them on purpose to intentionally work for you instead of unintentionally working against you. Teachers and parents sometimes say, "Watch your mouth, young lady/young man." That's what I want *you* to do: Watch your mouth. Be conscious of the power of your words. Don't use words and thoughts that work against yourself.

Become a Word Chiropractor

Complaining and negative self-talk create an energy that is completely counterproductive to helping you get you through your day. Using disempowering words and negative self-talk is an optimism buzz kill. I found it extremely hard to be optimistic when my palace pop-up pity party was having a picnic in my brain. What was the solution? I had to become a word chiropractor and make an attitude adjustment.

One of the fastest ways to get an attitude adjustment is to choose empowering words. The words I said to myself had a huge influence on my attitude, so I was careful to replace negative thoughts with positive thoughts really fast. How fast? Faster than a court jester can make a princess laugh.

It's not good enough to say you are going to press the delete button on a negative thought. You must have a positive replacement thought at the ready. Otherwise, you've created a thought vacuum that the negative thought can pop right into.

But that seems counterintuitive, right? I mean, let's just go after those suckers with an industrial grade vacuum hose. That approach won't work. Why can't we just stop thinking the negative thoughts? Because focusing on not thinking about them just makes us focus on them all the more in the same way that telling someone *not* to think of a pink elephant actually makes them *think* of a pink elephant. And if that happens, the only way to stop thinking about a pink elephant is to replace that thought with another. Have them think of a blue tiger, orange zebra, or magenta cow.

For example, if I had a palace pop-up pity party about my treatment, I didn't just tell myself to stop having palace pop-up pity party thoughts about my treatment. I used one of my princess positivity practices such as thinking *Yeah, but I get to live!* Or I told tell myself that even though I was getting chemo, I was lucky to have insurance paying for it. Or I thought about the fact that I had access to great doctors. I did a little chiropractic on myself and adjusted my attitude.

I used the same approach when I worried that the estrogen blockers would make my skin shrivel up and turn me into Princess von Skinisfried. Those estrogen blockers were going to keep me safe. I applied the yeah, but I get to live method. And as it turned out, my skin was fine. It didn't change at all, which led me to suspect that sometimes our attitude has more power than we think.

Here's a secret. Each time I get my estrogen blocker pills refilled, I write on the bottle "Youth and Beauty Pills." I'm watching my words and creating new ones. And I found new and resourceful ways to look at these potentially negative events in my life in positive ways.

Ditch the Labels "Good" and "Bad"

In addition to watching words, watch how you label circumstances. It isn't helpful to label what is happening good or bad because often, we don't really know if something is good or bad. Often, we're wrong, and it's both. Often what is happening is not an all-or-nothing proposition. Here's my version of a vintage tale that illustrates the point.

A long time ago—before there were dating apps and respectable bars—a beautiful young princess lived in a huge palace. She never went on a date because the king and queen were strict vegans and were waiting for the right person of like "prince"iples to court their daughter. She thought she might search for her prince in the local mall, but her parents wanted no courting in a food court, which would be kind of tacky for a princess.

The princess longed to meet a fine young man, yet it seemed that all the available beefcakes ate beef. And while her parents required her to be a vegan like them, she longed for an opportunity—even if just once in her life—to shimmy up to a counter with a tray holding a big, juicy burger with bacon, lettuce, cheese, onions, pickles, and ketchup.

One day, the beautiful young princess lost one of her favorite mares. All the townspeople came from far and wide to express their sympathy, but the princess held her head high and was totally chill.

Using negative self-talk is an optimism buzz kill.

A few days later, her mare returned, and beside her galloped a handsome stud. And he ate vegan-style!

The subjects were happy and came to congratulate the princess on her good fortune. But the princess retained her equanimity. "Joyfulness often brings tears, so who can tell me for sure that this won't turn out to be bad fortune?"

The beautiful princess and the young vegan-style-eating prince became fast friends. He loved to ride the wild horses from the king's stable with her. Unfortunately, he was thrown from one of the wildest of the horses and broke a leg. The townspeople came to share their dismay at the young man's misfortune, but the beautiful princess held her head high and said, "I reckon I don't mind this mishap too much. I know that good and bad fortune often live side by side. Who among you can know if this isn't a blessing in disguise?"

Not more than a few days later, big Blue Meanie invaders marauded the country. All the beef eaters of the land were told to join the army. The battle was treacherous, and sadly, many young men bit the dust. No more juicy burgers for them. But because of the vegan-style prince's broken leg, he was not sent to battle and was saved from harm.

The princess's parents were so thrilled, they allowed the princess to taste a big juicy burger with bacon, lettuce, cheese, onions, pickle, and ketchup for the first time in her life.

Whether that was good or bad is a mystery that has come down to us through the mists of time. To this day, no one knows on which side of the fortune fence *that* one lies.

The labels of good and bad have to go. Not only are they often inaccurate, they can hinder our finding the good that we search for in our quest for a positive mindset.

When I stayed over at my brother's apartment the night before each chemotherapy, I slept in the loft area. Above the bed was a window where doves nested. I loved to hear their soothing, cooing sounds in the early morning. No wonder they were the symbol of peace. In my mind, doves were very good. They contrasted with pigeons, which I certainly did not see as good. Pigeons pecked, littered, and crapped all over the place. In my mind, pigeons were bad.

As it turns out, doves and pigeons come from the same family, the Columbidae family. In fact, some pigeons are referred to as city doves. And the differences between the two family members are mostly in their physical characteristics. It's pretty much like many families— maybe even yours—where all of the members look pretty darned good but some are tall or short, blonde of hair or brunette, princes or princesses. Doves and pigeons are all one big happy feathered family. What can we learn from that? Drop the labels. It's all about how we see things.

I asked myself if it was possible to do the same with cancer. Could I eliminate the good/bad dichotomy? How could I possibly see cancer in any light other than bad? I discovered that I could. I remembered that everything is a plus. I just had to be on the lookout for what was good about the situation. I found a lot of good. For example, becoming more mindful of the present, role modeling how to handle challenging times for my kids, and finding meaning by helping others were all good in a situation I might have otherwise labeled as bad.

The key was that when I was un-labeling, I couldn't weigh the good and the bad against each other to see which had more weight. I couldn't just say that the bad of cancer was so much worse than the good of mindfulness that it outweighed the good, making it null and void. No! The good did count. I couldn't slap a concrete label on it because it was too dynamic for that. It contained both.

When I thought about it, I realized that I was labeling my estrogen pills in my mind as something bad. But that was ridiculous because they were saving my life. That's why I decided to write "Youth & Beauty Pills!" in permanent marker on every single refill bottle.

The less we label things good or bad, the less mental work we have to do to get around circumstances that pull us to label things bad. Easier said than done? Perhaps. But practice makes princess perfect. Now that you are aware of these issues, you have a foothold in mental toughness. You will ascend toward a higher rung on the optimism scale.

Feed the Good Wolf

Fanny taught me that thoughts are like a muscle. What you focus on strengthens, and what you let go of and don't focus on atrophies. In practical terms, when we focus on our positive thoughts, we strengthen them, and the negative, fearful thoughts naturally tend to whither.

Many of us know the old story attributed to the Cherokee about the two wolves. In that story, a Cherokee grandfather wants to teach his young grandson about life. "There is a terrible fight going on inside me between two wolves. One wolf is evil. The other wolf is good." The Cherokee grandfather then explains to his grandson that the fight between the good and bad wolves is not only going on inside him, but in everyone.

The little boy looks up to his grandpop with big eyes. "Grandfather, which wolf is going to win?"

"The one you feed," his grandfather replies.

We all must remember to feed the good wolf. When the evil wolf starts talking in your head, don't feed him. Don't feed the evil wolf that tells you you're not good enough, not brave enough, not strong enough, not attractive enough, not going to make it, or any other snotty "not." Instead, feed the good wolf. Focus on positive self-talk. Focus on the wolf that says you have the courage to meet the challenge, you're beautiful with or without hair, and you're going to make it. Sometimes the evil wolf will seem disproportionately hungry. Starve him and feed the good wolf.

Using positive self-talk instead of focusing on how big cancer seemed to me, I focused on the power that I had by just being alive. I focused on the fact that I was living and breathing—right then and there. I said to myself, "I am strong, I am healthy, I am powerful, and I am healed. I have doctors helping me every step of the way." I was constantly feeding the good wolf.

Learn to accept the is-ness of things, and the difficulties of life that you cannot control will be a lot easier to take.

By feeding the good wolf, we are not changing the facts, we are changing our focus and our magnification. We are magnifying the positive. It's a choice. It's a powerful tool among all the tools to which we have access for healing: mental strength to magnify our fortitude and resilience, the power of modern medicine, and our soul connection to serendipity and synchronicity. It's all good stuff, and I choose to magnify that good stuff—that wonderful good wolf!

I even feed the good wolf for my dog Lalo. She's an older French bulldog (a Frenchie). Every day I say this over her: "You're a young

Frenchie. You're healthy and strong. You are going to live a long time, all healthy and strong. Your youth is continually renewing, and so is mine." And then I say something I say to myself every day, three times. It is a shortened version of something Lucius Annaeus Seneca said a couple of thousand years ago. "Today will be the best (finest) day imaginable." I don't know why I say it three times. A princess idiosyncrasy, I reckon. But guess what? Lalo hasn't complained yet! I feel happier when I declare the health of my dog and help her feed the good wolf. Maybe she feels that good wolf is part of the family.

Every time I chose words that felt empowering about my treatment—whether it was referring to my chemo days as my spa days or telling myself that my radiation tattoos were angel kisses—I fed the good wolf. We get to choose how we look at life.

Believe it or not, all of this good wolf feeding truly helped me face the day. It ever so slightly, and sometimes hugely, took the sting out of the situation. It was kind of a chuckle and a wink, wink to my situation. Call it cancer jauntiness. It was a way of telling myself to lighten up. If I was actually going to die, I did not want the days I had left to be awful. I didn't want to be bluer than I had to be. I wanted to keep my eye on the prize: beating the breast cancer blues.

And I'd like to point out that I'm still here. I think that feeding the good wolf had something to do with that.

Find the Plus

You've already been introduced to Fanny, but there are a few things I haven't said about her experience on the run during the Holocaust. Fanny cheated death many times as she tried to get from France to Switzerland, and she told me many of those stories.

One stranger hid her in a coffin to help her get to another town. One young girl on a train shared her food and signaled Fanny to turn back from the town she was headed to because there had been a massacre there the week before. One family let her hide in their barn, only to turn her in for money. She was corralled onto a bus transport to certain death in the camps. All the victims were tied to their seats on the bus, but miraculously, Fanny's ties were not fastened. The woman sitting next to her draped her skirt over the evidence so the guards would not see that Fanny was not tied to the seat. At the next stop, the woman encouraged Fanny to run and escape, which Fanny did. So many of Fanny's friends and family were traumatized, and many were killed. But Fanny and her immediate family miraculously survived.

But here's the miracle that I want you to know, and Fanny would too. Despite all of this, despite all of life's woes, Fanny continually said, "Didi, *tout est un plus*," meaning, "Didi, everything is a plus." Over and over, this was her watchword phrase. Her mother taught her this, and Fanny continued to believe it as well. This was Fanny's *leitmotif*. When I think of her, I think of *tout est un plus*. She has saved me many times over with this pithy phrase.

The reason everything is a plus is because there is always something to be learned from any situation, something good that we can make of it as we move forward in our lives. Fanny's story is inspiring on many levels, including its lessons in resilience, in keeping going, and in having a wonderful life "in spite of." If Fanny and her family could continue to believe with all their heart that everything is a plus, then I could believe that everything was a plus too.

I searched my mind for ways to look at the situation with new eyes and to reframe what was happening to me as a plus. When I looked, I found there were many ways to see this experience as a plus. I spoke earlier about some of the pluses to having a mastectomy that I came up with. But there have been so many others. Making the decision to look at cancer as an adventure was a powerful plus because an adventure carries with it the possibilities of discovering new things about myself, meeting wonderful people, and having new experiences.

Another way breast was cancer was a plus was that it was a catalyst for finding another tier of meaning in my life through finding meaning in the breast cancer journey. And as I said earlier, I was able to be a role model for my children on handling the curve balls life throws at you. Being able to find deeper layers of meaning in your own life *and* model that for your children is about as good as it gets for a parent.

Another plus has been getting a chance to *live* my eulogy instead of having it spoken in my absence after death. Yep, that's right. I've felt the extreme, concentrated, heart-on-the-sleeve outpouring of love and caring of family and friends that many people won't get to feel in their lifetime. I got to have people find the courage to come up to me while I'm still alive and tell me all the things you hear at funerals! How's that for a perk? This has taught me that we don't have to—and we shouldn't—wait for people to keel over and die before we tell them the good stuff we feel about them.

Another plus is learning and relearning to deeply savor the present moments in a more intense way. I use the word *relearning* because bringing my mind to the present moment requires continued refocusing. As the brouhaha subsides and the exigencies of cancer fear mitigate, believe it or not, life normalizes. And life has normalized for me. I don't want to lose my pluses. To make sure of that, I draw on the experience of breast cancer to remind me, and re-remind me, that life is not a given. Every moment must be savored

By seeing everything as a plus, I was also ripping a page from Pollyanna's playbook by invoking the glad game. I am of course referring to the book *Pollyanna* by Eleanor H. Porter. Pollyanna took a lot of heat for her sunny disposition and dogged determination to find the bright side. She sought out the bright side by playing a life game her father had taught her: the glad game. If her father had been a positive psychology major, he would have understood that he was teaching her to reframe with that game. The goal of the glad game was to find something to be glad about in any situation. The cool thing about Pollyanna was that she used the glad game to help all the people around her. She didn't just use it for herself.

Think about that. If you take Pollyanna's approach, your positive disposition can be something that helps heal the world around you.

The word *Pollyanna* has been given a bum rap, but I'm here to reclaim her status as a brilliant happiness torchbearer. She was not a blind optimist. She saw problems but chose to do something other than focus on them. She fed the good wolf. It was a skill she exercised and taught others. Pollyanna believed that by searching for the things that make you glad, you forget the things that can make you sad. Sounds like Fanny's advice, to exercise the happy emotions and let the negative ones atrophy. For sure, Pollyanna knew about the other kind. She was orphaned and exiled to her aunt's house, for goodness sake. But the difference between her and the folks who made fun of her was that she chose to do something about the tough stuff. Fanny and her mother were doing the French version of the glad game.

Endless Opportunities

The opportunities for princess positivity practice are endless. You can even make it a find-the-hidden-treasure-in-the-picture game. It's not hard to find the pluses in life. Make a decision to play the glad game every day. Resolve to hunt for something to be glad about and write it down so you can refer to it on days you need a lift.

In fact, write down a few of your favorite old-fashioned sayings that help you gain perspective or calm your nerves. Keep them nearby. Refer to them whenever fear or worry creep into your heart. For me, wise sayings were like lifeboats in a stormy sea. And interestingly, they somehow helped the waters return to calm.

We all get into a funk sometimes. But princess positivity practices can not only get you out of them, they can help make your funk frequency occasional instead of ongoing. And that's one way to keep feeding the good wolf.

If your mind goes, wahhh, wahhh, wahhh, here's what you do.
Tell yourself, Yeahbut, yeahbut, yeahbut...yeah, but I get to live.

13

Princess Positivity Pointers for Getting Through Getting Bald

There's nothing better than being bald for discovering
one of your hidden assets.
–Princess Diane von Brainisfried

The funny thing about this cancer thing is that aside from the issue of . . . well . . . cancer, some aspects of the disease and treatment are harder for some than for others. For me, in addition to the difficulty of being bald, I feared frightening my kids and everyone around me who might see me. I was afraid it would be the most significant symbol of being sick. I was afraid it would make me look pathetic. Not only did I not want to be or look pathetic, I wanted to be and look strong. I was not looking forward to the challenge of baldness, and I was definitely looking for guidance about it.

What helped me from the start was looking at the heroes who showed us their bald heads on YouTube. That is the one time I recommend searching cancer issues on the internet. Well, that and the makeup tutorials. It was super helpful to see others who had dealt with their bald heads as a result of chemotherapy and were not afraid to share what they looked like. How eye-opening. And many of these courageous ladies gave tutorials on makeup and how to choose a wig.

After viewing several videos, I realized I could have courage too. And I might actually look pretty good rocking a wig. That gave me a lot of courage too. What was especially helpful was seeing, firsthand, how hard it was to decipher that those bald ladies were wearing wigs. They looked beautiful! It was even more encouraging when they took off their wigs and they still looked beautiful, even when they were bald. Seeing all of this "full disclosure" will help you be brave to do the big reveal to your friends.

Sherpa Sherrie recommended that I buy two wigs, one for daily wear and one for exercising. She recommended that I purchase them before I had any hair loss to avoid any more anxiety than necessary. She also recommended that I get my head shaved around the time the oncologist pegged that my hair would fall out so I wouldn't have to go through the process of watching clumps come out in my hand. That was truly fabulous advice. Note that this all applies only if you are not having some hair-saving device during your treatment, such as a cold cap.

I went into New York City with one of my besties about a month or so before starting chemotherapy. Not only would she be there for emotional support, she could also help me pick out the style and color of wig that looked best on me. The place we went was very experienced with people who were purchasing wigs because of chemo, and there was a private room to try on the wigs. We had enough lead time in case I wanted highlights or lowlights in the human hair wig.

The expert there advised me not to make a drastic change in my appearance with the wig because so many other changes were happening. That worked for me, but I have seen YouTube videos in which women said it was fun to play with different looks, so just be aware of those issues.

I tried to reframe my thoughts about my upcoming hair buzz and baldness as a beauty adventure.

My wig expert was wonderful and kind. He recommended that I stay with long brown hair. I got one with long brown hair, only better. The color was a little more auburn than my own hair, and that was a nice touch. If the wig got wet, it turned into beautiful beachy waves. If it got wet? That was unthinkable with my natural hair. With my own hair, I never went anywhere without some sort of hair protection against the rain. But liberation came with my synthetic wig. It was fantastic.

Some Strategies for Getting Through Getting Bald

Any woman facing the prospect of baldness needs some princess positivity strategies to get through it. I may be a princess, but I was no exception. Having been advised to take matters into my own hands instead of ending up with handfuls of hair as chemotherapy did its number on my scalp, I decided to have my head shaved. My girlfriend and I planned a fun day around the event. She reserved a table for us at an elegant restaurant so we could have a beautiful lunch after my shearing. It was a brilliant strategy of distraction.

I tried to reframe my thoughts about the upcoming buzz as a beauty adventure. I also tried to look at it as indulging in curiosity about what I would look like bald. Here's the funny thing, ladies. You might discover hidden assets you never knew about. Maybe you have a beautifully shaped head beneath that mane of hair. Now that would be an excellent asset!

Additionally, a strategy I used to face getting my head shaved was to practice gratitude. I tried not to focus on the fear. I focused on being grateful for the opportunity to rock a new look that I would never in a million years have tried on my own. Okay, that one was a stretch, but it was something. And I had gratitude for the wigs that would help me feel like I still looked my best. Not a stretch.

But what about avoiding baldness altogether? Aren't there cold pack hats that some people put on their heads to prevent hair loss? Yes, there are, and they may be appropriate in some situations. For a number of reasons, I did not even investigate whether a cold pack hat would be appropriate for me. You will need to do your own due diligence on this. Whether you can use a cold pack in an attempt to save your hair (or save some of it) is something you need to discuss with your health care team and insurance provider.

Whether you use a cold pack hat, wait for your hair to fall out, or have your head shaved, it is helpful to use reframing and gratitude strategies to face the experience and make the most of it.

There's No Way Through but Through

As a teen in summer camp, I went on an overnight camping trip along the Appalachian Mountain Trail. Halfway through the hike to our destination, we faced a narrow ridge with a steep valley to either side. I was petrified of heights. I froze. I couldn't go back because there was no one to guide me. My frozen-in-fear body told me that I couldn't go forward either. *There's no way through but through*, I thought. I got through with the help of the camp counselor. This insight became useful when I faced another mountain in the form of getting my head shaved in preparation for the baldness that occurs with chemotherapy.

Right before I had my head shaved, my friend and I held hands tightly while the hair stylist swiveled my chair around. If I had to bet, I'd bet that he probably did that so I couldn't see what was going on. If so, it was a good plan. I didn't have the nerve to peek at all during the head shave.

It was a little strange hearing the buzzing of the razor and feeling it sweep up and down my scalp. I couldn't help but notice the waterfall of strands coming off down the shoulder area of my cape and onto the floor. When the stylist was finished, he turned the chair. I braced

I had to be brave for myself, because there was no retreating.

myself and took one quick look to absorb the shock while I had my friend with me. My heart registered about a 4.0 on a Richter scale, and then the stylist plopped the wig on my head.

It was shocking to see myself bald, but I thought of Fanny and repeated to myself, "Watcha gonna do with that?" I had to be brave for myself because there was no retreating. I thought back to my hiking days on that mountain. Once again, I realized that there was no way through but through, so I made the decision to be brave. And that was that. Like my grandmother Lena, I would do what had to be done. Like my camp days, I also invoked the aid of a friend.

The person who buzzed my head told my friend that I had a nicely shaped head and looked good bald. I would never have known that if my head hadn't been shaved.

My friend and I had planned a nice lunch at a great restaurant in the Time Warner Center, and it truly was great that I had something fun to look forward to. There were tall windows overlooking the city, and it was a beautiful, sunny day. All through the lunch I pretended I was a movie star with my glam new wig and new look. That part was pretty cool—and very princessy. It was also very distracting for my mind in the best way possible.

The point is that it will be a lot harder for you if you make it hard on yourself. Focusing on losing your hair isn't going to be productive, and it certainly isn't going to help you get through. That all being said, allow yourself some time to cry if you need to. Take some time for a private palace pop-up pity party. This stuff is hard. This stuff isn't entry level Life Course 101. This is advanced. Just don't stay in your private pity party room too long. Get in and get out. Does it take some mental work and focus? Yes. But it's worth it.

When I purchased my wig, I had also purchased a few head scarves and an adjunct to my wig repertoire, an inexpensive thing-amajig called a halo. This was a rather ingenious hairpiece that was sewn onto a headband. It went around my head like a sweatband. It was made to be topped by a scarf, cap, or hat. This bad boy was incredibly comfortable in extreme heat as an alternative to the wig, which could be hot.

Walking through Central Park on my way to a chemotherapy session, I had a new sense of awe and inspiration as I looked at the Orthodox Jewish women wearing *sheitals*, which are wigs worn for religious purposes. They looked so glam as they rocked their wigs in the oppressive heat. I figured that if they could do it, so could I. Never mind getting through chemo, I was interested in looking glam in my wig. I went through about two halos and two synthetic wigs during the bald stage of my chemo career.

I also became adept at wearing just the right kind of scarf, and I learned about that when one of my teachers went through chemo as part of her own breast cancer journey. When she was getting through getting bald, I gave her two of my favorite head scarves. One was pretty, red, and plain cotton. The other was a colorful Pucci-type of print that was made out of a padded quilted-like fabric. She liked the padded scarf the best and wore it all the time. I came to understand why, both from her experience and my own. The padded nature of the scarf gave it a little more frame to the face in terms of height, so it didn't just lay down on the bald head. That made it look more like there was hair on the head. Because of her experience, I understood the qualities that a good chemo scarf needed. And now you do too.

It really does help to use the strategies of finding things to be grateful for and reframing things in a positive light. I made it a princess positivity practice to focus on being grateful that I had medicine to help make me get well, grateful for a support system of family and friends, and grateful that I had wigs and scarves. I reframed baldness into something positive: I often looked better with a wig than with my own hair. And with the wig, I always looked styled. I could be playful with it and try new looks. I could add drama with hats. And most of all, I never had to worry about frizz!

Buying and Caring for Wigs

Learning the care and maintenance of your wig is another instance where YouTube videos can be really helpful. I did not attempt to wash my human hair wig myself. I recommend scoping out a trusted or recommended hair place that focuses on the care of wigs. I not only had a synthetic wig, I had a human hair wig. A human hair wig is a big-ticket item, and you want people who know what they are doing to wash and style it. Styling a human hair wig requires different skills from styling hair on a head, and if someone does a bad job of it, the hair is not going to grow back.

As for synthetic wigs, I googled up the wazoo to find out how to care for them. There are special products for synthetic wigs. I bought them, but I also found some homegrown ways to care for my wig that worked really well. Here are some tips for washing synthetic wigs that worked for me. Take a bowl that accommodates your wig and fill it with water. Add a combo of baby shampoo and mix that with about a capful of liquid laundry softener. Gently wash the wig by squeezing it, and then let it soak for an hour or more. Then gently rinse it in a sink under cold running water. Be very careful with it. Don't comb through it, not even with your fingers, or you might pull out some of the fibers. In other words, don't try to detangle when it's wet. Make sure the water runs clear. Gently squeeze your wig to get out excess water, but don't wring it dry or twist it.

Let the wig air dry on a stand. Don't use heat to dry it unless you are absolutely certain the manufacturer says you can. I am not sure I would anyway. Make sure it is completely dry before you comb it. I learned from the pundits that combing it when damp or wet puts too much stress on the fibers.

Take some time for a private palace pop-up pity party. This stuff is hard. Just don't stay in your private pity party room too long. Get in and get out.

And there you have it! This should keep your wig great for quite a while. Now all you need is your beautiful tiara, and you will be ready for a night out in the kingdom with your friends.

Sherpa Sherrie told me how to go about this whole wig process and guided

me on where to purchase a wig. She picked out her wig before chemo started so it would be ready for her when she needed it. She shaved her head a few weeks into chemo to avoid the shock of losing her hair in clumps. I followed suit. That produced very little shock time. I kept thinking of concentration camp victims and how they must have felt. Their lives were in danger every minute, and they certainly didn't get to wear a wig. I was in a much easier position to face the experience. No one was trying to kill me. They were trying to *save* me.

Sherpa Sherrie explained that I might want to purchase both a human hair wig and a synthetic wig. That way, I wouldn't get my good wig all steamed up and ratty when I went to the gym. That's why I bought both. I ended up wearing my synthetic wig much more than my human hair wig because it was wash and go, yet still beautiful. And as mentioned earlier, I also bought a "halo" synthetic wig (open on the top and worn with a cap or headscarf) to have something more breathable and less hot on my head in hot weather.

I suggest bringing a friend with you for your head shaving (if you choose to do that) and for the wig selection and fitting. Having someone hold your hand through the head shaving can be comforting, and it's helpful to have another opinion during wig selection. Could you bring your spouse or another family member? Yes. But not only might it be a bit much for them to deal with, it might also be a bit much for you if you see any hint of worry or other emotion on their face.

Wigs are awesome, ladies. And because they are necessary as part of a treatment for illness, wigs might be paid for, at least in part, by your insurance. Look into the issue of insurance and get the ball rolling before you need a wig so you can get approvals squared away if you do have coverage for them. Do realize that some back and forth with your insurance carrier might be needed. Be patient with them, and if frustration begins to fry your nerves, invoke one of my favorite princess positivity strategies for dealing with frustration. Remind yourself that they are doing the best they can. In the last years of his life, my dad told me that it was best to get the word frustration out of my vocabulary, so this strategy is Dad approved.

Keep in mind that if you get everything squared away with insurance and it's too far in advance of when you need the wig, you might have to get reapproved. In my case, the approvals had a time limit. My advice is keep a file on your wig insurance issues, ask a lot of questions, and make notes about who said what on what date so you don't have to rely on your memory.

Believe it or not, I told myself that when my hair grew back, I was still going to wear my wigs because I was so happy with how they made me look. No muss, no fuss. As it turned out, I didn't wear them after my hair started growing in. I never thought I would wear my hair so short and be happy about it, but I was. Still, just having my wigs when I needed them was an incredible princess positivity booster. You might find that they are for you too. Let it be a part of permission-mindedness. Give yourself permission to let something as simple—and potentially as important—as a wig support you on the journey.

14

BYOB—Be Your Own Bestie

When sadness starts to get some traction, BYOB
(be your own bestie) with distraction.
–Princess Diane von Brainisfried

You may have thought the acronym BYOB means bring your own beer or bring your own booze. Well, that's one way to look at it, but we breast cancer survivors need a different kind of BYOB: be your own bestie.

"Didi, you have to learn to comfort yourself," Fanny used to say. My sister used to put it slightly differently. "People have to be their own mothers." That may sound hard to do, but I have a few tricks up my satin and velvet sleeves that work well for me.

You may have heard of the child-rearing theory called self-soothing. I believe it promotes the idea that you shouldn't pick up a crying baby right away (after you've checked her for hunger, a wet diaper, or other obvious problems) because a baby has to learn how to soothe herself. I never followed this practice with my babies because it used to break my heart to hear them cry. Well, that and the fact that there's nothing more annoying than the piercing cry of a whining baby. I don't let my dogs self-soothe either. I'm constantly picking them up or petting them when they whine. I'm a *total* doggy enabler. But my point is, if a baby can learn to self-soothe, so can adults.

I've talked about how I gave myself permission to be happy and healthy "in spite of" my cancer diagnosis. After a while, I realized there was another area in which I had to give myself permission: having inner peace. For me, inner peace is critical for my happiness. I believe that without at least some sense of inner peace, it's hard to feel like I'm in a healthy mental place.

Of course, a little stress is not generally a bad thing. Without it, we would all turn into one of those novelty store rubber chickens without a backbone. But I'm not talking about really small levels of generalized stress, like when you can't find the corkscrew for the pinot. I'm talking about the big stuff. You know when you're entrapped in its grasp. It's like the classic definition of pornography. You know it when you see it. With stress on steroids, you know it when you've got it. It's overwhelm on overdrive.

When I was diagnosed with cancer, not only did the big things like surgery or chemo bring stress, I also had the mind trips of fear that arrived in rivulets like rain on a windowpane. A few of the biggest stress offenders I dealt with, especially after my diagnosis, were rumination, worry, and negative thinking.

At nighttime, trying to go to sleep was often difficult because my mind entertained circling "what if" thoughts. What if it has gone from my lymph nodes into my bloodstream and bones? What if it got into my chest wall? What if I cut myself and get lymphedema? What if I get an infection when I'm on chemo and I can't fight it? What if they can't cure me and the cancer comes back? What if all this stress ages me like a two-term president? What if chemo makes me nauseated and I'm throwing up all the time? What if I freak out the night before my mastectomy?

At those times, I told myself that stress was a normal reaction, and so was having inner turmoil. Right as rain, you might say. But that wasn't the point. I wasn't worried that I was thinking or obsessing in an abnormal way. I just didn't want to be in that uncomfortable mental space to begin with. So telling myself it was normal didn't help. As a matter of fact, I would rather have been Abby Normal if that's what it took to be out of inner turmoil.

And then it dawned on me that I needed a permission trilogy. I needed to give myself permission to be happy, I needed to give myself permission to be healthy, and I needed to give myself permission to have inner peace.

It's crazy how magic happens once we make a decision. As soon as I gave myself permission to have inner peace, I had the wherewithal to employ tools and strategies I already knew to help me. I had tools for these circling thoughts, ruminations, and other bothersome mind-trespassers.

Circling thoughts are just not helpful, and if we catch ourselves entertaining them, we should stop. We shouldn't berate ourselves, just note that we are doing it and stop. When I did this, when I appealed to reason by remembering that circling thoughts were unhelpful and did nothing but upset me, it was easier to stop them. But I also knew from experience and from other learned folk that when we stop a habit, we sometimes create a vacuum. Because of that, I knew I wanted to have something positive handy to replace the circling thought.

I developed some princess positivity practices and pointers to help me quash ruminating and circling thoughts. Let's start with rumination, because it is one of my specialties, and by that I mean that I am really good at doing it, so I have to work hard at minimizing it. Rumination is the tendency to repeat thoughts—often negative and worrisome ones—over and

I needed to give myself permission to be happy, I needed to give myself permission to be healthy, and I needed to give myself permission to have inner peace.

over again. You might recognize it as the feeling of being overwhelmed and stuck inside worrisome thoughts that are running away with you.

The word *rumination* comes from what a cow does when it chews its cud. It turns the food over and over and over in its stomach. That's called ruminating. Cud sounds like crud, and that's fitting. When we ruminate, we're turning something, usually some negative experience and the emotional fallout, over and over in our minds to process and digest it. That's kind of like what the cow does, only with our thoughts. What we do is chew our thought cud.

Here's an example. When I was first diagnosed with breast cancer, we weren't sure how bad it was. At the beginning, it seemed not-too-bad, but as the tests came in, it started looking more than not-too-bad. The problem was, I didn't know where on the roulette wheel of looking-a-little-worse the ball was going to land. I started thinking about it, over and over. Was I going to die? Were they going to be able to do anything for me? How would I tell my kids? I have so much left to give, what am I going to do? Would I need a mastectomy? Were people going to run away from me? Would I be lonely? Would I be unattractive? Would I be throwing up in my shoes?

Now here's the funny thing. Our minds think that chewing thought cud is doing us a favor. Author and researcher Sonja Lyubomirsky explains that our minds believe that such inward-focused rumination on a problem is the way to fix what's going wrong and maybe even lead to happiness. However, research by Lyubomirsky, Susan Nolen-Hoeksema, and others shows that inward-focused rumination can keep you sad or make you even sadder. Such rumination causes other negative results too, such as impeding the ability to concentrate and fostering a pessimistic outlook on the situation.[13]

This makes a lot of sense to me. In other words, the mind believes that it's going to help us solve problems and life issues if we put on our princess tiara thinking caps and start doing the merry-go-round mind shuffle. Perhaps it seems counter-intuitive, but ruminating on our problems can actually make everything seem like it's going to hell in a handbasket. If you're trying to solve what's going wrong in your life, rumination can make it harder to solve the puzzle. Worse yet, if you're trying to see your problems clearly, rumination can bend the lens on your thoughts and present you with a negative view of what is happening. Ruminating can grab you by the ruff and ring a bad mood around you that circles for days.

In the movie *Bridge of Spies* (which is about the Francis Gary Powers incident), there is a Russian spy who appears to be just a nice, respectable, older gentleman—no one flashy. He has been caught and is facing prison and potentially even death. But he doesn't seem worried. When asked about this—and he is asked about this numerous times—he makes it clear that worrying isn't going to solve his problems. It seems to me the guy had a hot tip from headquarters about the rumination maneuver: It ain't gonna help.

You can see why it's super important to take stock of your thought style to see if you're prone to thoughts that look like yesterday's country breakfast . . . re-hashed. If you are, now that you know the dirty little secret about the downside of rumination, it would be helpful to work on lessening this tendency.

Strategies to Combat Rumination and Worry

Here are three strategies from Fanny that are remarkably simple but have helped me innumerable times when I needed to be talked off the ledge. The first one comes from something Fanny used to say to me. "Leave the thinking to the horses. They've got bigger heads." I often think of her words if I am worrying about a problem and am in a loop about it. Not only does it bring a smile to my face to think of her watching down on me, but remembering her words releases the problem from my mind. Horses *do* have bigger heads.

The next strategy Fanny taught that she used when she had circling thoughts bothering her was to recognize that her thoughts didn't always support her mental and emotional well-being. She could imagine almost physically getting away from them, letting them know that they couldn't bully her. She would say to these thoughts, "If you want to come in here, I'm leaving! I'm packing my bag and getting out of here!"

It's crazy how magic happens once we make a decision.

A third strategy Fanny taught me is one I like to think of as the "mother puts the sick child under her arm and just goes on" strategy. She taught me to look at worries and burdens as if they're a child who is ill. You wouldn't get rid of your child. You wouldn't leave your child. You would just tuck that child under your arm and keep going. It was good advice. I tuck my worries and challenges under my arm and keep going. For example, when I was diagnosed with breast cancer and worried that every little pain meant that it was spreading, I visualized tucking the worry under my arm and getting on with my life.

Here's another helpful tool for ruminating thoughts. I call it the Scarlet O'Hara hatbox trick. When worries and rumination start, create a mental picture of a hatbox and put the worries inside it. Then put the lid on the box, tie a big beautiful ribbon around it, and put that imaginary container somewhere out of reach—a high shelf in the garage, the attic, or anywhere else not easily accessible. Then, like Scarlet O'Hara, tell yourself you'll think about it later and assign yourself a time to think about the matter.

It doesn't have to be that day or the next one, just sometime other than the moment right after you've stashed the worries away. Tell yourself that when you go for a walk, you'll think about it. Or on Tuesdays in the morning. Or when you go food shopping. To the degree that our brains tell us we need to be thinking about things to figure them out, we can tell ourselves we will, just not now. We'll do it at another time, a time we choose. Then do that. Think about it at that time. This is another version of assigning yourself a time to have a palace pop-up pity party. And remember what my mother taught me. Things always look worse at night, or if you're tired, or if you are sleep-deprived. The morning rooster might bring a fresh perspective along with your sunny-side-up eggs.

If an onslaught of worries keeps coming, just continue to remind yourself that now is not the time to think about them. Tell yourself that your worries belong over in the hatbox until next Tuesday afternoon when it's your time to take them out and think about them. And when it is time to think about them, allow only a certain amount of time for it. If all else fails, remind yourself that a princess does not do thought cud.

The BFF buffer is another technique in my tool kit to calm my nerves. That consists of picking up your phone (or two paper cups connected by a string) and talking with someone trusted and empathic. Everyone should have at least one of these people in their life, and everyone should be one of them. It can be a friend or relative. And if you are really a curmudgeon no one seems to like, use that as your impetus to change. You are going to need at least one trusted friend in your lifetime.

What do I do when I need the thought police to quash a raid on my inner peace? I tell myself, "I'm the master of my mind! Who's in charge here?" Of course, I am. And so are you, princess. You are the master of your mind, and don't let the runaway thoughts steal your peace. You have something to say about it. Crush the attempted raid and keep your peace.

This next princess positivity practice can stop rumination and stress in its tracks. It's considered a mindfulness meditation. Mindfulness is putting your attention on the now. It is often practiced by focusing on one or more of your physical senses. I call this practice "smell the roses and blow out the candles." I was familiar with this powerful strategy to help combat stress and was delighted to find it written on the wall in the ICU ward of a hospital. One of the nurses told me they teach it to their patients all the time, and it's one of their patients' favorite calming practices.

It's a simple practice. Just breathe in through your nose (smell the roses), then exhale through your mouth (blow out the candles). If you're allergic to roses, you're screwed! No, just messing with you. Make it "smell the lilacs" or something. I like this practice because it's easy to put in your pocket and pull out when needed. And I love the roses and candles images. They are also very easy to remember.

Affirmations are also a good way to knock out ruminating thoughts. And they don't just send those thoughts packing, they replace them with positive self-talk. Positive self-talk—AKA affirmations—train the mind to think positively. Try it. Couldn't *hoit*. For example, to get a leg up on my day and set the right tone, I start out by giving myself a positive affirmation princess pep talk. A good way to remember it is to tag the practice with a habit that you already do, like taking a shower or brushing your teeth.

I like to say my positive affirmations daily in the shower, where I use a really lovely scented soap. That way, while my senses are already surrounded by the fresh water, scented soap, and the bright start of a new day, I invigorate my soul with positive thoughts that either reflect who I am or who I want to be. It sets a great tone for the day. I bet you already have some affirmations to pull out of your treasure chest as armor against ruminating thoughts if they pop up during the day.

I encourage you to create your own private princess affirmations that only you know, that are specific to you, and that incorporate your positive dreams and goals. Make one of them your good health. The positive affirmation that I say daily is perhaps two minutes long. It makes me feel invigorated, powerful, and happy. I'm pretty sure it's not just the soap. I start out different sections of it with something like "I am thrilled and grateful that I am . . ." Fill in the blank with a desired goal you are working toward, and you will be calling it into the focus of your existence.

For example, an affirmation could be "I am thrilled and grateful that I am healthy, happy, smart, loving, and forgiving, and I am at peace." Or, "I am thrilled and grateful that I am a happy, healthy, and successful nurse/doctor/social worker/psychologist, and I help people." Or, "I am thrilled and grateful that my family is happy and healthy, and we do many fun things together." The affirmations can be anything your heart desires for your life, yourself, and your world to be like.

Craft your affirmations in the present tense because the personal growth pundits will tell you that your subconscious mind does not distinguish between past, present, and future events. For example, don't say that you hope to become healthy and strong, say something like "I am full of joy and gratitude that I am healthy and strong!" Call it in as your current truth. What a great way to start the day.

In addition, the practice of meditation has been an incredibly powerful way to help me with ruminations by helping my mind stay at peace. At the very least, I know I have a technique to go to an inward place that's peaceful if the ruminations become too much. Meditation has the added benefit of helping to create more focus and clarity.

I practice a mantra-based form of mediation called TM (Transcendental Meditation), but there are so many other forms of mediation that are not necessarily mantra-based. You can do a little research and find a meditation practice that best suits you.

Another good practice that is an antidote to an uncomfortable state of mind is distraction. I use distraction to give my mind relief when I'm worried and my mind is spinning out of control. I used this technique one morning when I woke up in a sweat, feeling overwhelmed by a major house renovation. Why that should have thrown me for a loop at 5:00 a.m. I cannot tell you. This is not the stuff of life or death, my friends. And my mind knows that as well as anyone. I'm teaching this stuff, after all. But my heart wouldn't connect to that truth that morning. So be it. That's why there are princess positivity practices and pointers. That's why I'm building my trusty treasure chest of ideas for when the goblins come and try to steal my joy.

What did I do on that particular morning? I used the strategy of distraction to self-soothe. I went on my computer and I did some busywork creating folders, downloading PDFs, and printing the PDFs from an online course I had bought about marketing. I was basically organizing folders, but it took some concentration. By the time I was finished, the crisis of nerves had passed, along with the grey cloud. I wasn't totally my chipper self by the time I went down to eat breakfast, but I was a heck of a lot improved.

The laughing angels technique is another example of distraction— this one using visualization. It's an idea I received to calm my mind when I was getting radiation and I had to stay statue-still. If I moved, giant beams would go someplace they were not supposed to go, like my heart and lungs. No pressure there! To create a focus on something other than what was happening, I made up a little game called the laughing angels visualization. I visualized happy, smiling angels swirling around me. I liked to give each of them personality. One of them was funny looking, with twinkling eyes and two big front teeth. She led the others around in a comet of sparkling swirls. The angels served not only as a diversion for my mind, but a helping supportive strategy, like having a friend holding my hand. It sounds a little strange, but I guess one is never too old for an imaginary playmate. Whatever works!

Pretty much anything you do that is a distraction from your circling, ruminating thoughts is going to be helpful. Take an exercise class, go to a local art exhibit, do some gardening, look for a new recipe and cook it, help out at a food shelter, clean your castle, walk the dog . . . just do *something* that doesn't involve your grey matter so much. Distraction is a powerful princess palliative for helping to break the rumination cycle. And by the way, I've found that any time I help someone else, I feel much better, no matter what my stinkin' thinkin' is. Rumination is no exception to this regal rule.

Sleep

The fallout from too much worry and rumination is having trouble falling asleep. Some nights I felt a bit of terror creeping up the back of my neck like a spider. Spiders are creepy enough, let alone coming with terror. I admit, though, that sometimes when I feel this way, I think of the darling, friendly, and beautiful spider, Charlotte, from the children's book *Charlotte's Web*, and I feel a little better about the spider thing.

I have a few sleep tricks up my sleeve that will promote a restful night when you are having some trouble sleeping and counting sheep is out of the question because Farmer Fred put up an electric fence. The first strategy is called "the gift of peace." This fabulous practice came to me in a whisper one night when I couldn't sleep. I had been praying for help to ease my mind, and I didn't want to take a sleeping pill. The still, small voice deep inside came to me and whispered, *Give yourself the gift of peace.* That beautiful phrase was the magic bullet. After that, I slept like a baby—a baby without colic, that is.

Note a little adjunct piece of information relative to the gift of peace. The still, small, inside voice also told me that the gift of peace does not come with strings. It is not held back from you, contingent upon whether you think you've been a good enough princess to deserve Christmas goodies or whether you think you deserve a pile of coal. Santa doesn't care. When he gets to your house, he just wants to dump the load out of his sack so he, too, can lighten up and fly lighter. So if you feel you don't deserve to be able to sleep or you don't deserve the gift of peace, nip that bad boy in the bud. You are most definitely deserving. Sleep and inner peace are not only for the perfect. If they were, we'd all be walking zombies right out of something like *The Night of the Living Dead.*

If you beg to differ, first of all, stop begging. You are entitled to your opinion. But then, I would point out all the imperfect biblical people who are considered heroes. Some of them killed people so they could sleep with a super model. Think David. Some of them killed people who were meanies. Think Moses. Some of them argued with God. Think Abraham. Some of them tricked people using a hairy arm. Think Jacob. Some of them didn't treat Jesus so hot with selective memory. Think Peter. There's a whole lot more of these esteemed yet faulty beings in the Bible. Maybe that's the point. In our respective heritages, these imperfect giants were loved by God. Remember that the next time you are tossin' and turnin' because of your fallacies and foibles.

If your sleep starts to suffer from your fears and physical challenges during your breast cancer journey and you are becoming your own worst enemy, stop that. You are well loved. Period. Princess says so!

Here's another great trick for sleeping that I use all the time. My mother taught it to me when I couldn't sleep as a little girl. Some people call it progressive relaxation, but I call it the rag doll technique. Starting with your toes, feel every single part of your body, and feel yourself consciously relaxing them. For example, think of your toes and relax them so you're like a rag doll. Then think of your feet. Be like a rag doll and relax them. Then think of your ankles, shins, and calves. Relax them as if you were a rag doll. Work your way all the

way up your body until you get to the top
of your head. This is extremely effective
for relaxation. If you like, you can start by
visualizing a Raggedy Ann doll. Unless rag
dolls scare you the way clown dolls scare
me. Then don't do that.

*I tuck my worries
and challenges under
my arm and keep going.*

My sister taught me another sleep
strategy my mom taught her. I call it the worry bird sleep solution.
When my sister had trouble falling asleep because of worries, Mom
said that she was giving her a "worry bird" and that my sister should
put all of her worries on the worry bird. The worry bird would fly
away, taking all my sister's worries with her. What a great image! Why
not create an imaginary worry bird? It could be a heron, a flamingo,
a robin, a cardinal, or a bluebird of happiness. Or imagine something
wild and innovative like a multicolored, madras and polka dot parrot.
Whatever your worry bird looks like is fabulous. Then just strap those
worries on tight to your friendly little helper and up, up, and away—
there go all your worries!

Does it sound like I have a lot of sleepy-time tricks? I do. I invoke
what I like to call my Divine Mind in me autopilot practice when my
mind is a merry-go-round that won't let me settle down and sleep.
One night when this was happening, I realized that I could call on my
God connection or Inner Spirit Princess, whom I also like to call my
Divine Mind. I asked her to run the show for a while. She told me to
go on autopilot and rest my mind while she took over for me. When
I thought about it, I realized that she was always running the show
anyway—breathing, communication between synapses and cells,
cells replicating. My conscious brain has nothing to do with that!
My Divine Mind told me to let her do the thinking and put my mind
at rest. I was astonished at how relaxed I became. I fell asleep, and
all the chatter fell away.

I find this to be a very powerful sleep technique. You can substitute different names for Divine Mind. I also like My Miraculous Source, My Divine Diva, my Divine Energy Source, Inner Spirit, and Life Force. I suspect these are also terms for what many of us collectively think of as God.

A variation of the Divine Mind sleep strategy that is also very effective is what I call the unconditional self-love strategy. I repeat the following silently, over and over and over: *My Divine Mind sends unconditional love to me. My Divine Mind sends unconditional love to me. My Divine Mind sends unconditional love to me.* This is a wonderful and life-affirming way to fall asleep!

You can also combine some of the sleep strategies you like into a new sleep strategy. It's a kind of smorgasbord sleep strategy. You can change it up depending on what you feel like practicing. For example, I have combined one of the Divine Mind sleep strategies with the unconditional self-love strategy and the rag doll strategy. It works like this: *My Divine Mind sends unconditional love to me and through me, and my toes feel completely relaxed like a rag doll. My Divine Mind sends unconditional love to me and through me, and my feet feel completely relaxed like a rag doll. My Divine Mind sends unconditional love to me and through me, and my ankles feel completely relaxed like a rag doll.*

One more sleep strategy, and this is one Fanny used when she had trouble sleeping. It is one of my all-time faves. Visualize yourself being held in two big hands, surrounded by light. Imagine the safety, comfort, and love emanating from the hands and from the light. It's an extremely powerful image. It helps me feel safe and peaceful. And since this image came from Fanny, her power, spirit, and love are wrapped into it, spreading her essence, love, and empathy out to all of us. Now I bequeath and pass it on to you. Fanny would love that! For additional guidance to improve your sleep, check in with my good friend, a leading sleep expert, Nancy H. Rothstein, MBA.[14]

Collect Strategies

Choose some strategies for dealing with rumination and worry along with sleep strategies that resonate with you. Make a list of them. Post them, put them in a pretty journal near your bed, and carry them with you in your purse so they're handy for when you need them.

Make up your own strategies too, and collect strategies wherever you can find them. Yes, that includes collecting them from your colleagues, family, and bestie. But remember: BYOB. To do that, you need to treat yourself as well as your best friends do. Your best friends can't always be with you when you need comfort, but you can be your own bestie by learning how to comfort yourself and practicing self-comfort whenever you need it.

And here's a bonus. Like every good princess, you can share your collected strategies with others so they can be their own bestie too.

Visualize yourself being held in two big hands,
surrounded by light.

15

Hop-portunity

A wise woman learns from life's challenges. A really wise woman learns from the challenges of others and how they handled them.
–Princess Diane von Brainisfried

Some cultural myths are hard to let go of. One myth that has swirled around in motivational speaking circles for many years is the idea that the Chinese word for crisis includes the symbols for both danger and opportunity. John F. Kennedy even included this interpretation in speeches he gave in 1959 and 1960. Who can blame the motivational speakers for latching on to it?

It would take a Chinese linguist to explain what it is really all about, and I'm neither Chinese nor a linguist. But ask me if I care. I don't because often, crisis *does* bring with it both danger and opportunity.

Time and again, we hear that when a person hits rock bottom or is faced with some really hard challenge, it ends up being the best thing that ever happened to them or they turned it into a triumph. Heck, I need only look at my diagnosis of breast cancer to see the truth in this symbolism. Breast cancer = danger (to my health). Breast cancer = opportunity (to grow as a person, to model handling challenges to my kids, to write a book and get to help lots of people, and to meet some extraordinary people).

It's vitally important that you evaluate your life and find the ways that breast cancer is value-added. Where those places are, I don't just want you to lean in, I want you to jump in! I want you to hop in! I want you to find these "hop-portunities" and see them as transformational catalysts for a better life.

Another word for *transformation* is *metamorphosis*. When I was first diagnosed, the phrase "the new normal" was floating around in my brain. Was I going to have to adjust to a new normal? Meh. That didn't sound so great. But then I thought, no way! I'm gonna blow right past the new normal and go to mind-blowing life transformation. Miraculous metamorphosis. Time for beautiful butterflies. New chic haircut coming. Very French! New chic clothes I can wear with a smaller size breast: gorgeous strapless dresses, cute T-shirts. I'm going to rock it! I'm transforming, and I'm going with the flow of it! I visualized the symbol of a beautiful butterfly fluttering over gorgeous spring fields of flowers to help me feel renewed, beautiful, feminine, and youthful as I embraced new life adventures full of light and love, living intensely in the day.

I decided I was going to hold my arms wide open to the positive possibilities in the form of opportunities inherent in transformation. And by the way, the ancient Chinese philosopher Lao Tzu *did* say something positive about crises when he opined that every misfortune has good fortune hidden inside of it. Kind of sounds like that everything is a plus deal, doesn't it?

My seeming misfortune contained some good fortune when it came to my appearance. Before breast cancer treatment, I had what I like to call brisket hair. It was long, lush, brown, and thick. It had curls when I wanted, and if I applied heat, brute force, and the perfect product, it was sleek and straight. It was happy, frisky hair-with-body kind of straight. The kind that can get a good frizz up in humidity. The kind you hate when you're a teenager but later come to love—especially if you lose it.

> If you were a garden in which happiness seeds were planted, gratitude would be your mulch, fertilizer, compost, and rainwater. Gratitude makes your happiness garden grow.

At the end of chemo, the roots of my scalp sprouted hair like the green shoots of crocuses in the spring. After a while, I had the semblance of a "look," albeit one that was short, short, short. Upon seeing my newly bobbed-by-God hairstyle, a screenwriter friend of mine said I looked Gatsby-esque. Now, *that* was romantic. Others told me it was very chic and very French. I had no doubt Fanny would have adored it.

One of the plastic surgeons I was going to told me that it was his job to observe women and that this new hairstyle was a fantastic look for me. It fit my personality, and I no longer had to hide behind my boobs and my hair. Who knew? I never knew I was hiding, but I was willing to take the compliment in any form. Who knew cancer would bring such a perk?

In a trillion years, I would never have chosen to shorten my hair so drastically. But as it turned out, it was fun to rock the new look for a while.

Not only did breast cancer give me a new hairstyle, it gave me a new hair color. I had been a raging brunette all my life, and I loved it. There's something sultry about a brunette princess. But there's also something romantic about having lighter hair, which I had never experienced. Enter breast cancer to change all that. After chemo, my hair came in a light shade of . . . something. To avoid skunk root stripes, I decided to try a lighter color until my natural brown color returned—if it ever did. Lo and behold, people loved it. And I looked more like my blonde-haired, blue-eyed mom. Not only did my husband see it, but I looked in the mirror and saw her. It was very gratifying, and it was especially precious because my mom had dementia. It felt like I was seeing her reflected in me, and it reminded me that she was still here. I am sporting my original hairstyle and hair color now, but breast cancer gave me a reason to try something new.

Here's another fortune from misfortune: I can finally wear strapless dresses! That is unbelievably fun. As a princess, I do go to quite a few galas and balls, and I had never before been able to wear one of those sexy numbers with no straps or even spaghetti straps. And what princess doesn't want to wear spaghetti? Now I can wear almost any kind of evening dress. I also love those off the shoulder blouses that look so amazing on everyone. I have swimmer's shoulders, so I like the way they look on me. Could I have ever even thought of wearing them before? Impossible. Call this trivial if you want, but I think that being able to wear strapless dresses could very well be on the level of the profound.

And now when I go shopping for athletic wear, I can actually find a sports top that fits. I used to look at the racks upon racks of sports bras for ones that accommodated "racks." Forget the promises that they worked for all shapes and sizes. Not! I used to wonder if I was some kind of freakazoid because nothing, absolutely nothing, harnessed the locomotion from my breasts when I locomoted. The sports industry just does not have a clue. Now I can wear designer athletic tank tops, looking and feeling fabulous. And I won't bounce when I bounce. I can run, dance, and do all sorts of sports without holding my arms across my chest like an Egyptian mummy. Let freedom ring! Although not earth-shaking, this is a mini-fortune from misfortune.

These are just simple examples of how one can find the pluses, the "hop-portunities," if you hop right in, go with the flow, and look at the opportunities for positivity in the challenging changes. But there are three big hop-portunities to the breast cancer experience that are truly transformational: the hop-portunity to live more in the present moment, the hop-portunity to live with more moment-to-moment gratitude, and the hop-portunity to live a more meaningful life.

Hop-portunity to Live in the Present

Learning to live in the present moment is one of the biggest gifts anyone could ever receive. This is the gut level understanding that we must enjoy the present moment and everyone and everything in it. We need to grasp this concept in a way that is not merely a casual understanding, the kind that just sits in your head. It deserves a lightbulb type of aha—one where the head and the heart connect. Hot diggity dog! Cancer is one of the biggest gifts to help you learn to "relish" life, with or without the hotdog.

With that understanding on a visceral level, not just in our brains but in our bones, we realize how fundamentally important it is to be present in every moment. *Présent du présent*—present (gift) of the present. Today is what's important. Today is the big deal.

Having been diagnosed with breast cancer is a gift in so many ways, not the least of which is taking a step back from your life as it was to reevaluate how you might live it better in the future. One of those ways for me was to reboot my desire to live mindfully, in the present moment, so that it doesn't feel like I am spilling any of my life down the drain.

Today is a gift comprised of 86,400 seconds granted to us from some mysterious, celestial, nonrefundable, nonexchangeable gift registry. That seems like a lot of time, but we all know the reality of it. Time flies like a runaway train! There *is* something you can do, though. It's been my experience that the more attention you give to your moments, the more those moments seem to expand and slow down.

It helps to have a "time catcher mantra" to remind yourself to stay in a state of present awareness. The one I created for myself is "Be here now, princess." Feel free to rip it off. Or you might like to say something like "Be here now, beautiful." Just keep your phrase short and sweet so it's easily remembered and makes you feel good about yourself.

Hop-portunity to Have More Gratitude for Life

There's a very old idea—and I think it is even in Proverbs—that if you've forgotten the language of gratitude, you'll never be on speaking terms with happiness. A mountain of research shows that when we focus on thoughts of gratitude, we prime ourselves for more happiness and joy. The positive psychology pundits are pretty clear that gratitude is a component of your inner life that has many health benefits, both emotional and physical. You want to be happier? Ramp up the gratitude. It could truly help change your life for the better. Look at it this way: If you were a garden in which happiness seeds were planted, gratitude would be your mulch, fertilizer, compost, and rainwater. Gratitude makes your happiness garden grow.

"Well, land sakes, princess," you say, "what do I have to be grateful for? I'm dealing with breast cancer!" Listen, been there, done that. When we're hurting, sometimes it's hard to focus on what we're grateful for. But here's the secret: *Everyone* has something to be grateful for. If you at least try to focus on what there is to be grateful for, it can help you get out of the endless loop of feeling sad. Of course, we're allowed to feel sad and sorry for ourselves. No one would fault you . . . or me. But if I don't want to stay in that space, I am going to have to do something about it. Are you in or are you out? Period.

Even if you only feel slightly better, better is better than not better. Feeling better is a sliding scale from one to twenty, with twenty being the best. Even if you were a one and now you are a two, that's something to crow about. Because tomorrow maybe you'll be a three. And after that, who knows? There is some relief in going from one to two, and until or unless we can get to joy, it's relief we're going for. Relief will do.

Here's a little trick to help you shift to a grateful mindset to start you day right. Ignite your gratitude by taking a moment in the morning when you rise to visualize your life as a gift. Unwrap it every day and enjoy it. What is the polite thing to say when you receive a gift? You say, "thank you!"

On a trip to Italy, I learned the expression *grazie mille*. I love that expression. It means "one thousand thanks." I heard it everywhere. Hold in your mind those lovely Italian words, *grazie mille. Grazie mille* that I have been given the gift of another day!

We can also use the concept of *grazie mille* with the thousands of things we can say thank you for *during* the day. "Thank you that I have friends to help me through my day." "Thank you that my children and husband are healthy." "Thank you, thank you, thank you."

Being diagnosed with breast cancer was a catalyst for me to up my gratitude game. I have been practicing gratitude for a long time, but this experience put the practice on steroids. It's amazing what new eyes you can have when gratitude is at the forefront of your mind.

Consider keeping a beautiful notebook or journal in which you write down what you are grateful for. Some people refer to this as keeping a gratitude journal. And the habit of gratitude journaling can lead to increased happiness. That's what a lot of research concludes. I recommend combining that with your synchronistic events, so maybe call it a gratitude and marvelous miracles journal or whatever fancy and fun name you want to give to your fabulous journal of life. Review your journal on a regular basis to give yourself a happiness boost and stoke your spirituality.

Here's an idea to make it a little easier to motivate yourself. Start with only three things that you're grateful for. Then, if you'd like, continue adding more things to the notebook on a daily basis. It's so easy, even for the grumpiest among us. There's at least something you will be grateful for each day. If you do it at nighttime, it's a great feel-good bedtime ritual. It can set a wonderful tone for sleep, as long as you are not grateful for ripping someone a new one. You can even be grateful that you wrote in your gratitude journal.

Hop-portunity to Live a Life with More Meaning

If I were asked how living through breast cancer impacted my life in a positive way, I would answer personal growth, spiritual evolution, and the ability to live life with a sense of passionate purpose and meaning (or as I like to say, *passionate porpoise*, just for the fun of it).

I can almost feel myself hopping up to a higher level of my becoming. It's not just my next step, it's my leap into accelerated growth. I truly believe cancer has bequeathed me that benefit because of all the searching I had to do to mentally survive. The searching led to answers and changes in perspective that promoted higher stages of personal growth and an even more positive attitude about my life.

I spoke of Viktor Frankl earlier and his teaching that whatever happens, we have the power to control our attitude about it. In writing *Man's Search for Meaning*, I think Frankl's objective was to model for us the idea that under the most horrendous circumstances imaginable to man, we have the capacity to find meaning. Holding the perspective and attitude that what we are going through has meaning is what can make terrible circumstances more bearable.

Experiencing a life-threatening event can jettison your life into a crucible of learning. You begin to ask important questions regarding the meaning of life globally and on a personal level. What is the meaning of *my* life? How can I *create* more meaning? Do I have unfinished business that I must focus on? And does the little stuff that annoys me even matter?

The whole thing, from diagnosis to treatment, feels rather surreal at times. But as a part of that surreal feeling, I had a sense that the cancer event was an otherworldly gift. It felt like I was tapped for a new journey of personal growth that was part of my destiny. Being diagnosed with breast cancer seems to have accelerated the process. On the one hand, the journey can be scary. But seen with new eyes, it's certainly interesting, and it holds the promised potential of personal growth for you and others on your path.

The minute I get to help somebody else, that's a really big bullet in my happiness ammo belt.

I've been on a trajectory of creativity my whole life. Throughout elementary school and college, I was always writing poetry. Even when I still worked as a lawyer, I began writing screenplays and musicals, transitioning out of law to focus more on those projects, as well as on motivational speaking. Since my early twenties, I have gathered and written notes about life lessons. I have reams and file drawers of paper filled with my thoughts. Then it was my computer that became the recipient of those thoughts. From reams to bytes: good title for a book.

Being diagnosed with breast cancer brought me new eyes to appreciate life even more. I have a new sense of my destiny and purpose. It feels like I'm on fire. Not a day goes by that my fingers don't fly over the computer keys as some unknown creative source does the writing dance for me. Perhaps that happens because I can so directly see the connection between what I am learning through breast cancer and how I can help others in a relevant and important way.

I am wholly trusting the universe to point me in the right direction. Because of my experience with serendipity and synchronicity, I believe that those who need to hear what I have to say and those I can help will find me. This whole experience is connected to fulfilling my destiny, making my own personal legend happen. It's one of my hop-portunities to make a huge difference in the world.

But let's talk about you. If your authentic journey isn't writing, it might be touching the lives of others in a significant way that you would not have had the courage to do before. Maybe you will tell someone you love them—someone who really needs to know that. Maybe you will help someone believe in herself. Maybe you will break down barriers. Maybe you will start to paint. Or if you paint, maybe you will begin to paint more passionately. Maybe you will sing. You will see so many blessings when you see breast cancer for what it can be—a gorgeous, beautiful transformer.

Here's a little hint. The minute I get to help somebody else, that's a really big bullet in my happiness ammo belt. There's just something magical that's self-helpful when you help someone else. It reminds me of an old Chinese proverb: If you want happiness for an hour, take a nap. If you want happiness for a day, go fishing. If you want happiness for a year, inherit a fortune. If you want happiness for a lifetime, help someone else. I was blessed with having an expanded vision of meaning in my life because I can now help others with breast cancer. That was a profound manifestation of a meaningful life. And here's the shocker: If I could wave a magic wand, turn back time, and remove the breast cancer experience from my life, I wouldn't.

Having breast cancer can be a huge hop-portunity to shake the fruit tree of your life and let the ripe fruit come loose. Whether it's making a decision to pursue a new goal, find a goal, or just make a change in your life, it can be a big fat do-over.

I read an article about a woman who was in prison for harboring a fugitive who happened to be her husband. Not only was the experience of prison its own kind of hell, it was also traumatic for her to see the suffering of her young daughter because of her incarceration. The only way she survived the yearlong sentence was to find meaning in the experience. She dreamed of setting up an organization to help the kids of incarcerated parents, and that dream not only provided meaning, it also gave her the resilience to mentally survive. When she was released from prison, she established the organization. Everything is a plus, and meaning is a *big* plus.

Danica's Gift

Many people in my life have given me the hop-portunity to look at life through a different lens. Danica was one of them.

Danica was a beautiful thirtyish classmate who studied with me in an online course. Danica was in my class for four years. When my teacher, my classmates, and I first met her, she told us she had the life-threatening disease cystic fibrosis. Cystic fibrosis is a congenital disease that causes sticky mucous to build up in the lungs. Daily therapy is needed from birth. By the time we met her, she told us she had already lived well past her expected lifespan. In typical Danica style, she tried to put us at ease by telling us not to worry, she wasn't going to die tomorrow.

Danica was so young, vibrant, soulful, alive, and seemingly rosy-cheeked healthy that the seriousness of her situation didn't fully register to any of us in the class. The precariousness of her health didn't compute. Danica was famous for her sweetness and her smile. She always brought a deeply kind and loving perspective.

As time went on, when we saw Danica in the little thumbnail video that patched us all into the online class, she started to show up at each session wearing an oxygen cannula. Danica never, ever complained, even when she could not attend class because of her illness. She sometimes shared a few of her hospital experiences, holding that radiant smile all the while. Even then, I didn't comprehend how hard life was for her. How could this beautiful, rosy-cheeked classmate be in that much danger? It didn't seem possible.

One terribly difficult and sad day, our class found out that Danica had a major stroke. She'd had a relatively minor stroke a few months before, but she had managed to bounce back, although with complications. But she still showed up, class after class, with that iconic smile of hers. We were asked to pray for her, and there must have been a cacophony of prayers sent up to heaven. But our dear Danica angel passed away the next day.

Long after Danica's passing, I thought about how many more years on earth I have had the blessing to live that she didn't receive: almost thirty. That alone was a tremendous gift that I had been graced with, breast cancer or no breast cancer. It dawned on me that no matter what difficulty I might face in a particular day, be it frivolous or major, Danica would have *loved* to still be around to work through what I was facing. I thought to myself, holy cow! At least I'm alive to face those challenges. What a new way to see challenges: being alive to greet them!

I realized something, and what I realized is the basis of Danica's gift. Every single inhalation and exhalation I have is one more breath that Danica would have been abundantly grateful to take. Every single one of those breaths I take without even thinking about it— unlabored, easy, and free—is a breath that Danica would have made joyfully. Danica made me see with new eyes.

Danica had been unable to breathe without difficulty. She needed a lung transplant, which she never got. I now see breathing for the gift of life it truly is. Every single one of our breaths is a gift. When I wake up, I take three big breaths of air, in and out, and then say, "Thank you, Danica!" What is so unbelievably surprising to me is that even though I

Today is a gift comprised of 86,400 seconds granted to us from some mysterious, celestial, nonrefundable, nonexchangeable gift registry.

stared down death with a potentially life-threatening illness of my own, I still needed to be reminded how precious every moment—and every breath—is.

Andy's Gift

One of my most precious possessions is an essay sent to me by my good friend Andy, a highly respected and honored medical doctor. He was voted by his peers as a top doctor in New Jersey and the greater New York metropolitan area, and he was a man of brilliance, warmth, humor, and empathy. Andy passed away a couple of years ago from cancer. A year or so before he died, Andy wanted to show me the speech he was going to deliver as an honoree at a hospital gala I would also be attending.

Later, when I was facing down my fears after being diagnosed with breast cancer, I remembered Andy's words of wisdom. One summer while on the beach enjoying a fireworks display with his family, he became annoyed and distracted by the up and down bobbing of a balloon on a long string tied to a chair in front of him. He almost let this small balloon bobbing in the endless sky ruin the entire night for him. But he told himself to stop focusing on the balloon and enjoy the show. He realized that the balloon was a metaphor for his cancer and the fireworks were a metaphor for his life. It's up to us to live our lives to the fullest each day, no matter what challenges we face. We can't let our hardships and difficulties prevent us from enjoying each day.

Now that you have this bit of Andy's wisdom, my royal friends, let it be a prized possession for you too. Promise yourself that whatever the circumstances, you will never again let the balloon distract you from enjoying the beautiful fireworks of your life that are truly the important show.

Betsy's Gift

My friend Betsy was inspiring in so many ways. She was thoughtful, smart, kind, playful, beautiful, joyful, and full of life. Her eyes twinkled when she talked. I was always uplifted when I spoke with Betsy. She was a wise, loving person.

Betsy thrived one day at a time, after being diagnosed with ovarian cancer years ago. Sadly, she recently passed. One time when I wrote to her to see how she was doing, she wrote back saying, "Doing fabulously! I am now at the Jersey Shore readying our beach house for renters. Miss you, hope the same sun and moon we live under look as wonderful to you as they do to me. Love you!" That spirit of life and adventure in adversity really boosted my spirits.

Betsy believed that in the times of great anxiety over these ailments, we must comfort and reassure the body that it's going to be okay so it can be at peace. How do we do that? "You put the highest ideal of love in your heart," she explained. "That calms the anxiety and fear."

I love the idea of putting the highest ideal of love in my heart. She called it "in spite of" love. It's a choice of the heart. You're affirming a loving path for yourself, in spite of.

We have the hop-portunity to do that every day. So here is what I suggest you say to yourself: *Hey, self. I love you no matter what! Now quit worrying.*

Today is what's important. Today is the big deal.

16

Today, and Today, and Today

Now is the new "and she lived happily ever after."
–Princess Diane von Brainisfried

$\mathcal{M}$y dear royal friends, we've come to the conclusion of our journey together. I hope you've had a few laughs. I hope you've learned some things that will make your life easier and less fearful. And I hope you consider me a friend.

Before we say adieu here, I'd like to sprinkle some more princess positivity in your minds and leave you with some concluding thoughts and observations.

Magnifying the Spiritual

Way back in the beginning of the book, I told you about the many synchronistic and serendipitous events that happened during my breast cancer journey. Paying attention to synchronicities and serendipitous events has been an element of the spiritual part of my journey. It has been key. So here is a suggestion: If you get frightened over a medical report, I encourage you to do what I do. Magnify your spiritual thoughts, not your medical thoughts. That doesn't mean you should ignore your doctors. I just mean that you need to use your auxiliary power—your spiritual power—to help you deal with everything.

Here's what I do that you might want to consider doing too. I think of the many mysterious, life-enhancing events that feel like the loving arms of the universe. I magnify these signs and symbols of support by focusing on them and remembering them. It's a strategy that has been hugely helpful when I am in a whirl of fear. It can be for you too. As Princess Diane von Brainisfried always says, "If you want to be happy, don't focus on what's crappy."

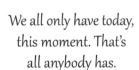

We all only have today, this moment. That's all anybody has.

God has you in the palm of his hand is an expression I love, and it happens to dovetail with the image I mentioned earlier that Fanny taught me to help me sleep. I imagine myself being held in two big hands full of light. In case you are not religious or spiritual, remember I am not without my own spiritual questions. We are in good company together. As Fanny used to tell me, doubt is a sign of an intelligent mind. But imagining yourself being held in hands full of light is a good tool for falling asleep—or comforting yourself, or quelling fear—whether or not you are spiritual, let alone religious.

They say there are no atheists in foxholes. Whether I believe or don't believe, whether I "know" or don't know, I feel something—an energy of some sort. Sometimes I feel it stronger than at other times. But I stoke my faith by learning about believing, by listening to what spiritual leaders have to say about faith. I listen to religious and spiritual sermons and programs. I read books on spirituality. I say affirmations of faith. As Fanny said, anything you exercise gets stronger, just like a muscle does. So I exercise my faith in those ways. Fanny also said that anything you don't exercise gets weaker, just like a muscle does. So I don't exercise my skepticism and doubts. I feed the good wolf.

What helps me have faith that the universe is supporting me and that Divine Energy is present are the miracles that I see every day.

This includes the signs and symbols I've been talking about. It also includes miracles we take for granted—the birth of a baby or a puppy, a sunflower field in the breeze, a ripe raspberry. I wake up to this reality. Hey, when you get down to it, it's *all* a friggin' miracle.

The wonderful, competent, and compassionate doctors and nurses who are here for us are also miracles. There's a miracle in the human spirit that nudges us to help and care for other people. I also focus on friends and family and the love we have for one another, the bonds and the ties. It's all a miracle. It's so mysterious, these emotional bonds we can feel but not see. And we feel them even when people leave this world to go to the other side. To me, it's like an invisible golden thread that goes from my heart to my loved ones in heaven. That is a miracle. I focus on everything that seems like a miracle to me, and in doing so, I magnify my spiritual side and not my medical issues. That always helps to calm me down and stay strong.

More than one lovely miracle of synchronicity has happened as I have worked on this book. Here's an example. You know what that magical time right before you fully wake up is like. It's a misty inner time when you're not really awake and not really asleep. It could be called *sleepwaking* (not to be confused with sleepwalking). It's when I'm in that state between sleep and wakefulness that I often hear bits of wisdom or feel that I'm communicating with someone who has crossed over. It's a time when I will often hear "inner-worldly" voices and ideas that seem to come from outside of me. It feels like I'm plugging into a greater energy or source to hear that stuff. It feels like someone else—or some larger energy—is whispering to me. I have come to call that energy The Inner Voice of the Sacred Space.

One Saturday morning, my radio alarm came on, and the music playing sounded like it was from the 1930s or 1940s. I was in that sleepwaking state when I thought about Benny, a classmate of mine from elementary school straight on through high school. I hadn't thought about Benny in years. In elementary school, Benny was a boy with meat on his bones, a crooked little smile, a gravelly voice, and a twinkle in his eyes. He was a good kid, and I imagine that his mom thought he was squeezable.

Benny was friendly and congenial, but he was also cool. I got a glimpse of this cool side of Benny when we were in fifth or sixth grade and I watched as a small crowd of kids gathered around him one sunny day on the playground at recess. Benny was aiming a magnifying glass at the toe of his leather shoe. All of sudden, smoke started rising, and when we looked closer, a perfect round hole the size of a cigarette butt had been burnt through his shoe. I don't know where the teachers were when this was happening, but God works in secret ways.

Unfortunately, I will never know more about Benny. He died in college. This was shocking news to all of us who knew him. He was among the first classmates of our youth to die.

That morning, when I was in the sleepwaking state, Benny popped into my head. Not only did he pop into my head, but I heard The Inner Voice of the Sacred Space tell me that there was a reason Benny popped into my head. And that it had to do with my book. I had no idea what the connection could be. I asked for clarification and went back to sleep. Howie had pushed the snooze button to silence the radio, so the radio show came back on ten minutes later.

And then it happened. The miracle. The synchronistic event. I heard something that made the phantom hair on my arms stand up. (I have no hair on my arms because the chemo took it away and it has yet to come back.) On Sunday mornings, a local radio broadcaster plays vintage shows. On one of those shows, two characters, a man and a woman, were having a conversation. I couldn't quite make out what they were saying. The woman was sobbing about someone named Benny. Finally, her sobbing subsided, and her words became distinguishable. She wondered if she would ever see Benny again. And then, her voice full of hope, she beseeched the listener to *bee-leeve*.

This was astonishing to me—so astonishing that I had to get up and write it all down. When I get messages like this, they are usually significant. If I don't write them down, I either forget them or I doubt that I heard them. I don't want the message in the miracle to get lost, so I write them down. As I mentioned earlier, to have a journal of these synchronistic events is a fabulous way to stoke your spirituality and suspend your cynicism.

> What helps me to have faith that the universe is supporting me and that Divine Energy is present are the miracles that I see every day.

I suddenly realized *exactly* how Benny fit into my book. It was a beautiful and clear example of synchronicity, a poster child for the "signs and symbols" from the universe guiding us, supporting us, and assuring us of our firm footing. This was a sign that I was so on the right path. Should we bee-leeve? Yes, we should.

Many mornings later, another message came to me to assure me that I was on the right track with my book. For some mysterious reason, I felt compelled to go over to a stack of old French fashion magazines that I had accumulated over the years to inspire me to keep up my French in a fun way. The fact that they were incredibly dusty should give you a hint at how well that technique was working. I randomly picked one magazine out of the pile. It was twenty-seven years old! I started flipping through the pages until I got to one that was dog-eared. I thought, ah, here it is. It was an article about families who sang together. There seemed to be nothing in the article that was relevant to my life at the moment, let alone the book I was writing.

For some reason, I flipped a few pages further, and there it was. In big, bold red letters was an article titled "*Optimisme, L'etat d'esprit anticrise.*" Translation: Optimism. The anti-crisis spirit. I saw it as another encouraging synchronistic event showing me that I was on the right track with my life and my writing.

And here is my final example before bidding you adieu. I had been asking Fanny to send me a sign of encouragement about my book. Although I almost always feel her energy and presence, from time to time, I want some worldly reassurance. I may be a princess, but I am also human!

I wanted to connect with Fanny really badly, and I felt so clearly that something was coming, but I had no idea where to look or what form it would take. As I was driving home from a doctor's appointment, I saw an elegant and sleek black sedan directly in front of me. It was just slightly too far ahead of me to make out the words on the license plate. But what I thought I saw had me smiling. I drove as close as I could without creating danger, but I still couldn't make out the letters for sure.

Finally, I got close enough to the back bumper to see the plate clearly. In bold capital letters, there it was—my sign from the universe, my sign from Fanny. The license plate on the big, black, elegant car read a word that I had heard Fanny exclaim hundreds of times when she greeted me: MADAME.

My Prayer for You

My prayer for you is that whatever your circumstances, may you find the desire to find happiness, may you make the decision to find happiness, and may you do what it takes to be happy. Joy is your birthright, and if you let cancer steal your joy, then you will have already died before experiencing the time you have left. Don't do that to yourself, and don't let your loved ones watch you do that. We all only have today, this moment. That's all that anybody has.

If you are in pain, my prayer for you is that you will be relieved of your pain and that you find comfort and happiness in whatever connections and smiles come your way each day and in the smiles you give to others. And I pray that you do not give up hope for a better day.

I pray that you will remember Danica's gift: gratitude for every single breath we take. If you are still breathing, you are still alive. If you are still alive, you have everything in this moment.

I pray that you will remember that every day, researchers come up with breakthroughs and new ways to heal and cure. And even if you believe there is no hope, there always is. There are always miracles. This world is full of mystery. The body-mind-spirit connection is full of mystery, and there are countless examples of "hopeless" cases that mysteriously turned around.

My royal friends, I pray that I have made a difference in your life for the better and that you can go out and help make a difference for the better for someone else. I hope I have served you well, that I have addressed some of your needs and concerns, and that I have helped you with some of your fears and worries. We are all in this crazy, fabulous world of experience together.

Remember, each of us only has today, this moment, and nothing more. Nobody has a guarantee about tomorrow. Today is as good as it gets. And it is royally good indeed.

My prayer for you is that whatever your circumstances, may you find the desire to find happiness, may you make the decision to find happiness, and may you do what it takes to be happy.

Acknowledgments

*H*ere's where I get to sing the praises of the many people in my kingdom who have made me royally happy and helped me along my journey of healing and thus must take some credit for the materialization of this book.

In addition to my beloved and very special parents to whom this book is dedicated, it is with incredible gratitude that I acknowledge the following people. My amazing husband, Howie, your love and strength helped me stay strong when I felt weak and fearful, your smarts helped me think when I was fuzzy, and your words always made me feel beautiful, even when I was battered, bald, and breast-less. Thank you for everything you've done for me since, including the animal crackers!

My wonderful sons, Harry and Max Uniman, you weathered the storm so bravely, and you'll never fully realize how that helped me weather it too. Thank you for that. I love you to the moon and back . . . and you always deserve it. To my dear in-laws, Joe and Shirley Uniman, although you passed before my breast cancer journey, thank you for your endless love and boundless support. My Aunt Sylvia Rosenthal, your humor is legend and you're a shining example that laughter is the best medicine. My brother-in-law, Charlie Uniman, you were a big support to me going through this. My fabulous daughters-in-law, Amanda Dillman Uniman and Liz Luckenbill Uniman, thank you for caring so much. You are adored additions to our family, and you both make family life feel like a party. Fire pit of truth. Hhuzzah!

Baby Joseph Uniman, you had me at hello, even though you can't talk yet.

Thank you, my brother, Carl S. Young, for being there in a big way from the starting gate. You always seemed to know the right next step. Your endless hours of researched analysis and reasoned guidance were a source of comfort and relief. I know you are not a doctor, but you could play one on TV.

My sister, Nancy Young, you *are* a doctor, and you continue to amaze me. Thank you for running interference when my mind couldn't grasp what was happening. I am ever grateful for your brilliant mind and street smarts. Thank you for the hours and hours of hand-holding and for always being there when I need you to help my worries fly away on Mom's Worry Bird. You will always be my beautiful sister. My brother-in-law, Jeff Melin, MD, thank you for offering terrific medical advice and supporting my creative sparks.

My extended family, Gale and Mark Dillman, Teresa and Craig Luckenbill, and Deb and Rich Ketner, you came into the family with warmth and affection. You made me feel that a big net of love was underneath me, so I could not fall. Moreen John, you are family too and you know it! Thank you for your loving support and words of wisdom during my cancer journey.

My professional colleagues who helped me get this book up and running—my Royal Cabal—I owe you so much gratitude! The trust we built up between us was something amazing. Cheryl Callaghan of The Author's Assistants, your breadth of publishing and marketing knowledge was incredibly helpful. You never missed a beat, even when I missed them! You kept it all rolling, and I am so grateful. Melanie Mulhall of Dragonheart, you're an editor extraordinaire. I think you might be a magician. Nick Zelinger of NZ Graphics, you're the cover and interior design king! You knew immediately exactly how to capture the dream. Big thanks to Karen Peters, my brilliant voice teacher, for the years of training so I could continue to fly and for the joy as you helped me work on songs I could include in my seminars.

I have had miracle-worker doctors and health professionals at many fine medical institutions. At Sloan Kettering Memorial, I am eternally grateful for Dr. Larry Norton. That's how you spell genius. Thank you so much for your brilliance and funny banter. You granted me my three wishes like the genie in the bottle: a chance for life, a chance for life, and a chance for life. Dr. Deborah Capko, you did a mighty fine setup for my new pair! Love our checkup chats. Dr. Peter Cordiero, you are an artist as well as a surgeon. My mirror, my clothes, and my psyche love you too. Dr. Mario Lacouture, thank you for taking care of the other areas that needed taking care of when chemo messed with them. Karen Drucker, thank you for bringing that smile with you every time I saw you, and thank you for laughing at my jokes. You went far and beyond duty, like finding my contact when it got lost in my eye. Thank you, Nickki Hamilton, for your easy way with the Prolia shots and your breezy way with conversation. Thank you, dear Sinead McCarthy, who always walked me in, for always knowing where to look for me and for keeping my spot in the doctor queue. And to Chaplain Clio Pavlantos, I send a big hug. Your blessings and prayers always came at the right time, and luckily before I fell asleep from the pre-chemo infusion!

At Fox Chase Cancer Center, Philadelphia, Dr. Kathryn Evers, you could have easily missed the tumor because it was really tough to see even on the 3-D mammo, but you found it. Gratitude does not even cover it. And an unbelievably huge princess bear hug to Cara Kowalski, whose proactive measures probably saved my life.

At Einstein Medical Center in Philadelphia, I give a heartfelt thank you to Dr. Lisa Jablon. Thank you for your brilliance, guidance, and good instincts that were always right. Dr. Corrado Minimo and Dr. Alessandro Bombonati, you are my heroes for your incredibly hard work. I am so lucky that you were there to help. You are also on my Big Pile of Gratitude list for your incredibly hard work.

At Robert Wood Johnson University Hospital in New Brunswick, Dr. Larry Haffty, thank you so much for everything you've done for me. The radiation technicians get a big shout-out too. You were so kind and fun to be around.

I would be remiss not to give a big shout-out to Dr. Gloria A. Bachmann for asking me to be the optimist expert at the Women's Health Institute. Your extraordinary talent and spirit go far beyond the technical side of medicine. And a big thank you to Amy Papi, of Women's Health Institute Advocacy/Community Outreach, whose unfailing support of my mission is a beautiful thing.

There were so many other doctors, nurses, and support people behind the scenes who were key to my cancer survival and good experience. Although I cannot know you all personally, please know that I am grateful to you. Although you and some of the doctors, technicians, and nurses mentioned here may no longer work at these institutions, you made your mark.

I also want to give a big, continuous high five of gratitude to the other health care professionals who have taken care of me on a routine basis. In particular, Dr. Carmen Tadros, Jim Gaido, Dr. David Shear, Dr. Thomas, Magliaro, Dr. Roshni Gandhi, Dr. Debora Goldstein, Dr. Mark Glasgold, Dr. Prapti Shah Chandrani, Dr. Alan Goldberg, and Danielle Shargorodsky. I appreciate you and how hard you work to keep me in tip-top health. But I also appreciate how much you care. And I appreciate your caring staff.

There are other folks I want to acknowledge who helped me on my journey. Amy Kernahan, of Amy Kernahan Studios, I am so grateful for your artistry. Wish I could hang out with you more! Stylists Edward and Barry Hendrickson's salon Bitz-n-Pieces in Manhattan, thank you for helping me find the perfect wigs. And thank you for helping me feel beautiful before and after the buzzcut. Nicole Campagna-Conway, thank you for always "getting" me and my hair and for doing everything in your trickster bag to transition me back to the me I want to be.

Carol Viscomi, your calming voice and practical advice eased my anxiety countless times and made the whole experience immeasurably better. Paying it forward is my gift to you. *Grazie mille, mille, mille per tutto!*

To Fanny Trueherz in heaven, I miss you, I miss you, I miss you. Your friendship remains foundational and your inspiration continues beyond the beyond. You show up in my life continuously. Words are not necessary. You understand all eternally.

Sean Griffin, you are a brilliant mentor and great friend. I can't wait to continue up the mountain with you and my classmates.

A thank you also goes out to Denise Ozoroski and Leslie Tietjen at Life Time Fitness. And thank you to Ned Webber of Phoenix Fitness. All of you have been instrumental in bringing me up to snuff on my physical health after the storm and helping me work around the challenge of no more "pec" work or downward dog.

Finally, I want to acknowledge how grateful I am for the additional members of my family and my dear friends, whom I love and who love me back. You know who you are.

Endnotes

1. Martin E.P. Seligman, *Learned Optimism: How to Change Your Mind and Your Life* (New York: Vintage Books, 2006), 15.

2. Seligman, *Learned Optimism*, ix, 14, 175.

3. Steven M. Southwick, MD and Dennis S. Charney, MD, *Resilience, The Science of Mastering Life's Greatest Challenges* (Cambridge: Cambridge University Press, 2012), 8-13.

4. Rick Hanson, PhD, Hardwiring Happiness: *The New Brain Science of Contentment, Calm, and Confidence* (New York: Crown Publishing Group, 2013), 23.

5. Seligman, *Learned Optimism*, 5.

6. Scott M. Peck, *The Road Less Traveled: A New Psychology of Love, Traditional Values, and Spiritual Growth* (New York: Simon and Schuster, 1978), 256-57.

7. Bronnie Ware, *The Top Five Regrets of the Dying: A Life Transformed by the Dearly Departing* (Macon, Georgia: Hay House Inc., Reprint Edition, 2012), viii, 167, 183.

8. Victor Frankl, *Man's Search for Meaning* (New York: Beacon Press, 1959), 97.

9. Frankl, *Man's Search for Meaning*, 98-99.

10. Norman Cousins, *Anatomy of an Illness*, (New York: W.W. Norton & Company, Inc., 1979), 43.

11. Patrick J. Skerrett, "Laugh and Be Thankful—It's Good for the Heart," *Harvard Health Publishing* (November 24, 2010),

https://www.health.harvard.edu/blog/laugh-and-be-thankful-its-good-for-the-heart-20101124839

12. "Laughter Therapy Shown to Boost Immune Function," *Medical Bag* (May 27, 2014), *https://www.medicalbag.com/lifestyle/laughter-therapy-shown-to-boost-immune-function-in-cancer-patients/article/472627/*

13. Sonja Lyubomirsky, *The How of Happiness: A New Approach to Getting the Life You Want* (New York: Penguin books, 2007), 112-113; 327 Note 41.

14. Nancy H. Rothstein, MBA, *The Sleep Ambassador®*, *www.thesleepambassador.com.*

About the Author

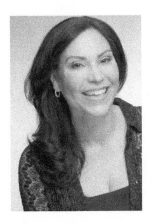

When Princess Diane von Brainisfried is not smashing champagne bottles over the bows of ships or blogging her brains out at her palace desk in the kingdom of *www.princessdianevonbrainisfried.com*, she's a motivational speaker and Certified Positive Psychology Life Coach. She recently put the rubber to the road and her money where her mouth is, having kicked breast cancer's arse without losing her happiness mojo. Her humorous seminars and workshops employ strategies for living your royally happy, radically fulfilled, richly meaningful life. Princess Diane is also the optimist expert for the Women's Health Institute of Robert Wood Johnson Medical School, and she was a facilitator at Miami's first World Happiness Summit.

When the princess is not wearing her tiara, she is known as Diane Young Uniman, a Phi Beta Kappa graduate of The University of Pennsylvania who also studied at La Université de Poitiers, La Rochelle, France. She's a criminal justice appeals attorney turned writer of screenplays and musicals. Her work has been featured at Lincoln Center's Broadway's Future series and was accepted into Fringe/NYC. She has won over fifty awards for her screenplays and musicals.

Diane is also an opera singer and an advanced student at the New York School of Practical Philosophy.

If you would like to follow Princess Diane's adventures and insights, you can do so at the following:

www.princessdianevonb.com
www.facebook.com/princessdianevonb
https://twitter.com/princessdvonb
http://instagram.com/princessdianevonb
https://www.youtube.com/princessdianevonb
https://www.linkedin.com/in/diane-uniman-bb548635/
http://www.pinterest.com/princessdvonb

The princess is also available for speaking.
Contact her at *princessdianvonb@gmail.com.*

CPSIA information can be obtained
at www.ICGtesting.com
Printed in the USA
JSHW010739290120
3874JS00001B/2